Intermitten Women

A Complete Guide to the Intermittent Fasting Lifestyle: Get the Clarity You Need for Rapid Weight Loss by Intermittent Fasting on a Ketogenic Diet

By

Jason Moore

Table of Contents

Introduction

In our society, not one day goes by where we are not bombarded with images about what our ideal body shape should look like, what we should eat, wear, and ultimately how to diet. It can be exhausting trying to keep up with the latest diet fads or even what the new size zero is.

But what if you did not have to conform to society's ideal and crazy beauty standards? What if there was a combination of diets that worked so well you would be at your target weight in no time? Did I mention that you would also stay at this target weight?

Dieting should not be about the latest fad or newest size triple zero, but about what you are comfortable in for your body, what you need, and what you want to see in yourself. There are healthy weight ranges that you should always strive to be in order to be your best self. And I have the world's best-kept secret on how you can do that!

One diet might sound crazy, let alone tying two diets together. But stick with me on this crazy train, I promise at the end of the ride your dieting life will forever be transformed. As women, your goals will all differ depending on what you want to see happen to your body. That is okay. That is why this diet combination works so well. Instead of putting everyone on the same diet and giving them the same goal, this diet can be shaped to match not only your lifestyle but also your individual goals.

You might just want to have a healthy average weight. You might want to pair this with a workout regime so you are fit, and you might even have a goal of having the hottest summer body out there. If these dreams seem impossible to you now, soon they will be within your reach. It does not matter what your end goal is, if you put in the work and stick to your diet then I guarantee that you will see results!

No, this is not another gimmick. Before you roll your eyes and put the book down, give me a chance! Here, let me explain some more. As a woman, you have a busy schedule, and your life is filled with a million and three different tasks for you to do. Keeping up with another diet might just seem like too much of a hassle for you. But what if that diet becomes a lifestyle change and habit?

Intermittent fasting is not just starving yourself. When you use intermittent fasting, you get to choose your own cycles in which you decide to eat and fast. So, it is all on your schedule! Sounds like heaven, right? A way that you can effectively diet and fast based on times that work for you! Maybe even a little too good to be true. But I promise you it is all possible!

Intermittent fasting alone does not restrict the kinds of food that you can consume, and while it is still effective this way, it is best when paired with the ketogenic diet. Together, these two diets keep your body in its optimal metabolic shape that will help you lose and burn all that excess fat you do not want hanging around. It also has other health benefits! I will go into more detail later about why these two methods of dieting combine so well together, and how they boost your overall results.

Weight loss is about more than just having the perfect body shape and size. It is about your personal journey to discovering how you see yourself. Your outside body is just a reflection of who you are on the inside. You can utilize intermittent fasting to help get you to your goals, maintain your goals, or even surpass your goals as you set new ones! This journey can be about your health, your weight, or just for your own peace of mind with yourself.

Intermittent fasting can help you lose weight, improve your overall metabolic health, and it can even help your immune system and protect you from other diseases! It may seem impossible at first to separate times that you eat from times you do not. You are most likely used to methods of dieting that involve snacking throughout the day. The great thing about intermittent fasting is that there are several different ways that you can merge it into your life. So, it is entirely possible to find the perfect method of fasting that fits into your schedule.

Think about this: there are already 8 hours of the day where you fast. When you sleep, you are not eating. This period of time is calculated into your fasting time, so you already have 8 hours down! Now you just need to decide where the other hours are going to come from, and since there are so many different ways to this method of fasting the possibilities are almost endless. I know it might seem scary to restrict your eating times at first, but when done safely and correctly people often report that they experience more energy than before they started intermittent fasting. There are lots of reasons for the burst of energy you will experience from this dieting technique, and we will get into all these in depth later in this book!

If you are worried about hunger, starvation, and any other combination of weird symptoms while starting this diet, I have one word for you – RELAX! Intermittent fasting is not starving yourself! And intense feelings of hunger are usually only felt at the beginning stages of the diet. Like with any changes in life, there will be a transition period. Be graceful with yourself. Give yourself leeway to make mistakes, but remember what your end goal is and commit to doing better the next round. This diet is about finding what is right for you and what works for you.

Everyone's journey will be different. And it is okay if your journey does not look like your friend's. All that matters is that you are on this path for yourself and your health. I look forward to starting this journey with you and guiding you through the steps and information you need in order to optimize your dieting methods.

Chapter One: All about Intermittent Fasting

History of Intermittent Fasting

Fasting is not a new concept. In fact, the odds are you have probably heard about it in many different instances throughout your life. Typically, you might hear it tied to religious practices. Perhaps you have even heard of intermittent fasting and passed it off as a new fad based on older traditions from past generations.

The truth is that intermittent fasting is about as old as humans. Yes, ancient civilizations used methods of starvation in order to keep their bodies in ultimate shape and reap the health benefits that fasting offers. They knew a lot more than we give them credit for, and we still use their knowledge today!

It did not matter where in the world our ancestors were located, almost every ancient group had a method of fasting or starvation that allowed them to obtain health benefits that included treating certain ailments, and even preventing diseases. Yes, you read that right! Our ancestors used fasting methods to prevent themselves from getting sick.

You might have heard of Pythagoras. He was an ancient Greek philosopher. You read that right: ancient. Seems like a different world ago? Well, that's because it was a different world back then, but that did not stop Pythagoras from boasting the benefits of fasting and encouraging those around him to do it.

Fasting has been in all aspects of our history. From health benefits to religious reasons, and even for political measures. Remember Gandhi? And the suffragettes? They fasted in order to illustrate how serious they were about their causes.

Mind-blowing, right? Well, it did not stop with our ancient ancestors. Throughout time and history, fasting methods have been used to strengthen bodies and immune systems. From ancient times to the middle ages, last century, and even in current times fasting has been used by the people of the world. There are many people today who reap the benefits that fasting has to offer.

Some people do it out of religious beliefs. Religious fasts date back centuries and occur over a vast variety of religions and cultural beliefs. But from these religious practices, their bodies are rewarded with a host of health benefits. There are even studies being conducted and published that indicate a direct correlation between the benefits of fasting and longevity of a lifespan.

Recently, intermittent fasting has gained more popularity. That is because it works! You might have thought it was just a fad or another passing diet. In fact, you might have thought that the diet just came into fashion for it to go right back out again. I have some news for you. Intermittent fasting has been here for centuries and will be here for more to come. And it all comes down to the bottom line – people experience amazing health benefits when they fast intermittently.

Yes, fasting has also played a role in the dark side of history. Keep in mind that fasting horror stories and the extremists that you hear of are not fasting correctly! There is a safe and proper way to fast. Depriving yourself of all food is not the way to go, and not what I will teach you in this guide.

Intermittent fasting has long been a part of our history as humans. As long as we have existed so has fasting. There have been countless studies done – even more recent ones – that illustrate the health benefits that intermittent fasting can provide to you. I promise I will go over all these benefits.

Will Fasting Work for Me?

As with anything in life, there are some people that think intermittent fasting is simply not compatible. It is important to know your limitations and if you and fasting are a good match. Sometimes it can be hard to discern if a new lifestyle change is right for you, and that is why I provide some helpful information for you to make an informed decision.

There are just some people who should not try intermittent fasting, and that is okay! There are other methods out there that might fit your needs. Intermittent fasting is a serious lifestyle change to add to your dieting methods, and so beginning this change needs some serious thought.

If you have ever or are still suffering from any kind of eating disorder, then intermittent fasting is not for you. It is important to know your limitations, and unfortunately, this is a limitation for those who have suffered from an eating disorder. Intermittent fasting can serve as a trigger for those who have or are suffering from disordered eating. And your health should be your number one priority! That is the premise of intermittent fasting, and sometimes you are at your healthiest when you are not restricting your eating times.

Restricted eating times and calorie counting prompts someone who has suffered from an eating disorder to fall back into old habits and patterns. Make sure to talk to your doctor if you think that intermittent fasting could help you, but you have had trouble with eating before. They will be your best guide to navigate this situation.

If you have type 1 diabetes, this might also not be the diet for you. Regular meals are needed to keep your blood sugar levels happy if you are a type 1 diabetic. With that being said, it is not impossible to fast intermittently while being a type 1 diabetic, but it is strictly recommended that you consult your doctor before making any dietary changes. As a type 1 diabetic, your bodily functions are in a delicate balance, and you would not want to unnecessarily upset that balance for a diet that will not work for you.

Intermittent fasting is great when it works for you, and since it is versatile, it can fit into many different lifestyle schedules. But if you are pregnant, then you should not fast. There are various reasons for why you should not fast while pregnant, and a vast majority can be discussed with your physician. One of the main reasons is that it can negatively impact your growing baby. There have been studies that also indicate long periods of fasting can impair your child's learning abilities later in life. So, while intermittent fasting has amazing health benefits for you, it is a no-no while pregnant!

As a woman, your body is constantly going through changes, and hormones are no stranger. But there are some things you need to consider before you take the plunge into intermittent fasting. Intermittent fasting can have many effects on your body, and I will dig into the meat of that later on in this guide. But one of the main things to take into consideration is if you have a menstrual period. It is not recommended that women who suffer from amenorrhea – otherwise known as the lack of a menstrual period – to fast intermittently. Fasting intermittently will already bring some changes to your body, one of the initial signs for women is a lack of a period. So, if you already miss your monthly period, then intermittent fasting can cause more issues with your system and how it regulates.

Always consult your doctor before making a big lifestyle change. Especially if you are concerned about how intermittent fasting might impact a health issue you are going through. The diet offers amazing benefits, but sometimes it is just not for you. It is always better to be well informed and at the top of your health game!

Fasting Myths

As with anything in this world, there are myths that surround fasting. Some are unpleasant myths, some are over the top, and some even promise unattainable goals. Put on your myth-busting gear because we are about to blast through some common myths!

It can be easy to get caught up in the glamor or horror story someone is telling you. And when you first start telling people you are trying intermittent fasting, there is bound to be at least one person with a story to tell you. It can be hard to wade through what is true and what is just extra noise in the dieting world.

One of the most common things you will hear about fasting is that skipping your breakfast will make you fat. Breakfast has been regarded as one of the most important meals of the day, and many people inaccurately assume that, by skipping breakfast, you are setting yourself up for failure. This is not true. In fact, there was so much debate about this that a study was founded, and it showed that there is no difference in weight gain or weight loss between individuals that ate breakfast and individuals that skipped breakfast.

Eat frequently, and your metabolic rate will be increased. Ah, the age-old fable that eating more frequently will help you lose weight quickly. This is largely dependent on the number of calories you consume, not how many times you eat. So, the bottom line? Eating more frequently does not burn more calories than eating less frequent meals.

What about the hunger myth? You have probably been conditioned to believe that eating more frequently also helps reduce hunger cravings. Well, I am glad to bust this myth. There is actually no real evidence that snacking more reduces hunger cravings. In fact, the findings of studies done have been varied. It almost always depends on the individual. And if you can get through the first stages of making a lifestyle change, the odds for reducing hunger cravings are in your favor with intermittent fasting.

Have you ever heard that if you eat smaller meals more frequently you will lose weight? It is really simple. If frequent meals do not boost metabolism, and they do not stop hunger cravings, then there is no way they can prompt you to lose weight faster than other dietary methods. Meal frequency has no effect on weight loss, so whether you eat three meals a day or six, you will not see much difference. That is why intermittent fasting is so different! Because instead of focusing on meal frequency you will be focusing on a window of time where you can eat.

There are also myths that fasting is bad for your body. Nothing could be farther from the truth. As you will learn from reading, intermittent fasting has a pool of amazing health benefits for your body and mind. It has even been proven to increase your lifespan. So, block the nay-sayers out and focus instead on what scientific results have brought you – intermittent fasting is a good thing.

For the grand finale, one of the most common misconceptions you will hear is that fasting will put your body into starvation mode. What is starvation mode? Well, starvation is when your body is pushed to the point that it shuts down its metabolic system, and as a result, you stop burning fat.

This is not true. As with any weight loss plan or dietary plan, there comes a point where you have lost so much weight that you do not burn as many calories as you first did. This happens with any weight loss diet, not just intermittent fasting. Short term fasts have even shown an increase in a person's metabolic rate!

Who Benefits?

I am glad you asked! I know I might have scared you a little with the "intermittent fasting might not be for you" talk. That is just because it is important to be informed, and making an informed decision is far better for you!

For those that intermittent fasting cannot help, it is unfortunate. But there are still a wide range of people that intermittent fasting is perfect for! There are benefits to this, after all, otherwise, you would not be considering doing it. Intermittent fasting can actually work out for a lot of people, and millions benefit from it year-round. So, by now you are probably wondering: "Am I a good candidate for this?"

If you do not fall under any of the categories mentioned above, then great news! Intermittent fasting may be an option for you. Mom with a busy schedule? Kids keeping you busy? Work always has you running around? Long lazy days at the beach? No matter what your lifestyle situation, intermittent fasting can benefit you. Even better, it can fit into your crazy schedule – no matter what it looks like. Choosing this lifestyle change all comes down to the individual. Intermittent fasting can work for you, but it needs to be done correctly. Often people pair fasting intermittently with an exercise plan or another diet type in order to get the best results from it.

You might still be unsure if this is the right move for you in your dieting career, and that is okay. You can consult your doctor to be sure that intermittent fasting is a good match for you. Keep in mind that there will be an adjustment period, but the benefits will far outweigh the cons at the end of the day. Keep on reading if you are still sitting on the edge of that fence! Finding out about how intermittent fasting really can be sustainable for you might just make you hop on over that fence.

Why is Fasting Good for Me?

I am glad you asked! Now we can get a little more into detail about those amazing benefits that intermittent fasting provides. I am guessing that you must be just a little tired of me going on and on about how amazing intermittent fasting is, but holding back on all the detail. And there is more detail to tell. But I will give you a brief overview, just so you know what kind of diet partner you are contemplating dancing with.

Remember my boasts that intermittent fasting can lengthen your lifespan? Well, it turns out those were much more than just mere boasts. Evidence has indicated that intermittent fasting changes the ways that our genes, hormones, and other cells function. What does this mean for you? Well, your body is going to undergo changes. This means that the regular way you produce energy needs to shift. It shifts from using your glucose levels to accessing your stored fat.

That is a pretty big change for your body to undergo, and it relies on other smaller changes to occur as well. The changes in your genes and the removal of waste from cells is what promotes a longer lifespan, as well as the disease prevention that I mentioned earlier.

Of course, the primary goal for many people who start intermittent fasting is to lose weight. Losing belly fat in particular and other unwanted excess weight is another benefit that people seek from intermittent fasting. The overall goal of intermittent fasting is to shrink your eating window. When you stick to your fasting schedule, your growth hormone levels will increase, and your insulin levels will go down. These changes, coupled with additional levels of norepinephrine in your system, increases the breakdown of your body fat for energy use.

Norepinephrine is a hormone that your body uses in order to regulate blood pressure. It works as a neurotransmitter. That is another reason why intermittent fasting can work for people who have low blood pressure.

If you are worried about your risk for type 2 diabetes, then intermittent fasting might be just the thing you need in order to get your body back on track! One of the changes your body will go through are lower levels of insulin. This is good news for type 2 diabetics as high levels of insulin are a cause of concern and worry.

Ever heard of the term oxidative stress before? If you have, you know it is not something you want to experience. For those that have not, oxidative stress is essentially the first step toward aging and other chronic diseases that you want to prevent. Intermittent fasting has been proven to reduce oxidative stress. See? Disease prevention at its finest when you let the body do what it was made to do!

Your heart is the primary vessel of your body – other than your brain of course. Your heart is what keeps blood pumping from each little finger to each little toe. So, it should come as no surprise with all the other benefits that fasting has to offer that your heart is also included. Heart health is an amazing benefit from fasting! Your heart health factors in so many different aspects from blood pressure to blood sugar and even body inflammation. Because fasting can improve all these factors, it has a positive outcome on your heart health levels. Our ancestors really knew what they were doing, right?

I mentioned the brain just above. Another one of our highly important vessels that we depend on for deeper levels of thought, introspection, and communication. Our brain acts as one of the lifelines of our body, and therefore what is good for our body is great for our brain! So, all those lowered levels of blood sugar and insulin, lessened body inflammation, and that lowered blood pressure positively impacts the way that our brain functions. It's like giving our brain superfoods!

These benefits are just scraping the surface of what intermittent fasting can really do for you. So, if you are already blown away by how much it can improve your health, hold on to your seat because there is more.

How Do I Fast?

Intermittent fasting works great because you are not restricting yourself from all eating, just limiting yourself to eating during a certain timeframe. There are several ways that you can go about accomplishing your goals.

When you look up fasting methods, you will see three main popular ones pop up. There are different ways for you to adapt this to your life, but I will go over the popular ones too. After all, there is a reason they are the most popular – they have been proven to work time and time again.

The most common method that people find manageable is the 16/8 method. The 16/8 method would mean that for 16 hours a day you fast, and the other 8 hours of the day you can eat! Relax. If you are freaking out about not eating for 16 hours straight look at it this way, for 8 of those hours you are supposed to be sleeping. So really, you are just splitting the rest of your waking hours between eating and non-eating.

Most people elect to do this by skipping breakfast. One example of the 16/8 method would be where you start eating at noon and stop eating at eight o'clock at night. It really does work, and if you have a busy schedule, you might find that there are already many days where you do not eat for a period of 8 hours.

Some people do what is known as the 5:2 method. This involves eating regularly for 5 days of the week, but for two of the days, you restrict calorie intake to only 500 calories. It is another popular method as some people do not feel like they are restricting their eating window too much.

The third diet that has hit mainstream popularity is known as the eat-stop-eat method of fasting. This way of fasting includes a full twenty-four hour fast. What this means is that during the week you set aside one or two days (depending on what works best for your lifestyle and goals) and you do not eat anything from dinner one night to dinner the next night. This can be a harder diet to maintain as those with impulse control, and snack habits can find it hard not to eat for twenty-four hours straight.

There are other fasting methods as well, and I will go in depth with you later in this guide. Intermittent fasting is not about cutting out all your food, but rather limiting your eating so that you can discover the best version of yourself. Mind, body, and soul!

Time to Check In

Phew! Okay, so well done on making it to the end of chapter one. If you feel a little information overload right now, do not worry. I am right there with you. I know I just threw a lot of information onto your plate, and it can take a minute or two to digest what it means.

Because it was so much to take in, I just want to make sure that the key points from the chapter stuck with you. So, in order to do this, I will just briefly go over the highlights. This way I know the most important details are fresh in your mind!

- Intermittent fasting has been in practice for as long as mankind has existed. It is not a new term or brand new diet fad – in fact, it will be here for as long as mankind continues to exist.

- There are a lot of myths surrounding fasting. It is always good to be well informed and know fact from fiction. Your friends might be well-meaning when they give you a fact about fasting that you know is untrue, but it is only because of all the misconceptions about fasting that exist.

- Knowing how to safely fast is the key to success.

- There are some people who are not a good fit for fasting. If you suffer from type 1 diabetes or even a lack of a menstrual cycle, you might want to put serious thought into a different type of dieting method. Always consult your doctor.

- Intermittent fasting can work for a lot of other people, though, and that is awesome! It has some seriously great health benefits that you would be remiss to skip out on.

- Fasting changes hormone growth, gene processes, and has been known even to increase the longevity of your lifespan. A longer life and healthier living options? Where do I sign up?

- If you are trying to avoid type 2 diabetes, fasting decreases blood sugar levels and can be an indispensable asset to you along the journey.

- There are different ways to fast. It is important to find what works for you. Not everyone will fit into the same box, and that's okay! That is one of the reasons intermittent fasting is so great – because it is so versatile.

In the next chapter, we will really go more in-depth into why intermittent fasting works, and how it really can work for you. It is a big lifestyle change, but there are tips and techniques that can make your fasting journey easier. If you have lasted this long, then what are you waiting for? Turn the page and dig into that next chapter of information.

Chapter Two: Fasting and Losing Weight

It is A Relationship

Intermittent fasting and weight loss are in a relationship that needs balance. As with any diet, stability and a plan are helpful when trying to stick to your goals. The main reason most people start fasting is so that they can lose the weight no other diet has helped them to lose yet.

Yes, fasting can provide a host of other benefits. But sometimes you just want to look like the best you externally, because that is the you that you feel like internally.

And let me be clear. It is completely okay if you are fasting to shed those pounds. In fact, it is awesome! Your journey to the best you that you can be just got one step better. Armed with the knowledge from this guide, I am confident that you will not only reach your goals but that you will conquer them.

There is a huge difference between fasting and starving. And sometimes when you need support from those around you about fasting, their first instinct is that fasting is starvation. It can be helpful to explain to them what the difference is and where the benefits lie.

Starvation is nothing close to fasting. During starvation, a person is involuntarily deprived of food. They have no idea where their next meal is going to come from or when it is going to come. Fasting is a controlled method of eating only during an allocated time frame. Your body is not starving, you are not starving, and you know exactly when you are going to eat next. It is a completely voluntary process, and you have complete control over it.

Losing weight comes with its own set of health benefits, and those are some health benefits that I am sure you are excited for. And I am excited to see you realize your body dreams and goals come true.

It should not be about an unhealthy relationship with food. I want you to love eating, and enjoy it when you do eat food. And that is why there is a crucial balance you need to maintain when intermittent fasting. You cannot revert to a period where you are always in fast mode – that is unhealthy, and you will then be forcing your body into starvation from depriving it of nutrition.

Intermittent fasting is a great tool that you should know how to access and maintain – regardless of what your final goals are for it. Remember, our ancestors have been benefitting from these methods long before we were even a spark.

How Do I Lose Weight?

Remember when I talked about your hormones? Well, that has a lot to do with losing weight while fasting. The main goal of intermittent fasting is to change the way that your body makes and uses energy.

I am sure you are familiar with the regular cycle of glucose from your high school biology class. And if that class is a little fuzzy, all you need to know is that your body likes to use it for energy. But this is not the only way that your body can produce energy. Yes, you read that right. There is more than one way for your body to produce and use energy.

Your excess body fat is merely your body's own storage system for energy – or in other words: calories. When you fast, there are three main components that change in order to start converting that stored fat into the energy you need to function. These changes all have to do with your metabolism, and that is why fasting is a great tool for aiding weight loss, everything always comes back to your metabolism.

Your insulin levels are one of the first things that will change. The more you eat (especially carbohydrates), the higher levels of insulin your body will produce. However, when you automatically reduce food consumption, those levels of insulin drastically drop. This is where fat burning really begins.

Your body also produces a hormone known as the human growth hormone, or HGH for short. HGH does a lot for your body, but for our interests, we are really interested in two of the things it helps out: weight loss and muscle gain. Because who does not like being toned? When you are fasting, it has been proven that your HGH levels will drastically increase.

And finally, the third component for your metabolic change is norepinephrine. Yup, there is that pesky long word again. Remember, it just acts as a neurotransmitter! This is the key part in converting fat to energy as the nervous system will use norepinephrine to begin breaking down body fat into fatty acids. These fatty acids play a crucial role in your energy needs.

Intermittent fasting is essentially putting your body into short-term periods of fasting, and there are many studies that prove that short-term fasting increases your metabolism. This, in turn, increases fat burning. See the cycle coming to life?

Calorie counting is important in any diet where you are really trying to lose weight. While it is not at the forefront of intermittent fasting, it is still important to be aware of how many calories you are eating.

Despite fasting, in your window of time when you are allowed to eat you still cannot overeat. If you overcompensate for the hours you did not eat you will do more harm to your body than good. All those good benefits you worked so hard to get will be flushed down the drain.

Intermittent fasting naturally works well because most people end up consuming far fewer calories in their eating period than they would if they ate all day long for sixteen hours.

A big concern for some people whose diet is the loss of their muscle mass. And that is the unique thing about intermittent fasting. Because of the way it works, you are more likely to maintain your muscle mass than lose it. Studies have proven that fasting has helped people retain or lose less muscle mass than they do on other conventional diets.

The overall change that aids your weight loss is simple. You are using your body fat to produce energy for your daily functions. And with that, you are inviting a host of other health benefits as well!

Intermittent Fasting is Simple

At the end of the day, intermittent fasting is a very simple method.

While there are a host of variations that you can use in order to fit it into your schedule, the concept is fair and easy to understand. Restrict your eating times, do not overload on calories, and maintain a schedule.

Fasting this way also promotes a healthier diet. If you are conscious with your food choices, your weight will be gone before you even know it. There are a few things you want to pay attention to and monitor when you decide to intermittent fast.

Do not slack on the quality of your food just because you eat for a shorter duration of the day. Food quality is extremely important. Whole foods should be a number one priority. They are better for you overall. In the next chapter, I will go more in depth about the foods you eat and what to try to avoid when intermittent fasting.

Consistency is key. Keep up with the schedule you set. Maintain your goals and standards. Like with any new change there will be an adjustment period, but if you can make it through that, then the rest of the journey is quite literally a breeze. New habits eventually become old habits.

I have said it before, but it is important, so it bears repeating. Do not slack on your calorie counting. While it is not as important when you are fasting, it is crucial that you maintain a balance. Overcompensating on calories will do you and your waistline no justice.

Patience is a virtue. But with a dietary and lifestyle change, you will need to practice this virtue. Be gentle with yourself and give yourself some time to make the change. Adapting to an entirely new way of thinking about dieting and food can be challenging. Your body will also go through changes, and in the beginning, they might not all be pleasant changes – we will discuss these changes soon. I promise you it gets better and it gets easier.

Time to Check In

There is always a lot to take in when making changes. So let us just recap what this chapter really was about:

- Intermittent fasting is a good safe way to lose weight.

- It helps increase your metabolism.

- Insulin levels will drop, growth hormone levels will increase, and your body will be told to start breaking down your stored fat into energy.

- Stored fat is broken down into fatty acids. These are then used for energy in a cycle called ketosis. It is opposite to the glucose cycle.

- Intermittent fasting is still a big change, so give yourself time and be patient.

Intermittent fasting works best when it is paired with another popular diet. This diet is called the Ketogenic diet. You might not be familiar with it, but by the end of the next chapter, you will be. You will also begin to understand why the ketogenic diet and intermittent fasting work better together than any other diet combination out there!

Chapter Three: The Ketogenic Diet

I know. More talk about diet! You picked this book up and thought it was all about fasting. Trust me here, it will all make sense in a bit.

Remember when I was talking about the importance of eating healthy? Well, the ketogenic diet is a diet that highlights whole foods and healthy foods. That is why the keto diet and intermittent fasting go so well together, like a fine wine combination.

The ketogenic diet is another diet that has become extremely popular in the last few years. But, much like intermittent fasting, people have been using the keto diet for many years. It actually gained popularity for a reason totally unrelated to losing weight.

This diet focuses on bringing your body into a state called ketosis. It changes the way your body uses and produces energy – just like fasting does. The premise of the keto diet is that it is a high-fat low carb diet. I know it can be shocking to think about since most diets consist of a high carb low-fat basis. However, carbohydrates raise your glucose and blood sugar levels. If there is an influx of glucose in your system, your body will revert back to producing energy for your use through glucose. And what we want is for your body to use your stored fat for energy, not glucose.

The focus of the fat portion in a keto diet should still be on whole healthy fats. There are plenty of fats that are healthy for you! When you eat a diet that is high in fat, you are giving your body a constant supply of energy, and this is why many people on keto report to feel energy increases when they make the change.

When you are making a choice to start the keto diet, you need to also switch the thinking that you have been conditioned to believe. Fats are not bad for us. Our bodies need fat in order to function, but there are differences between unhealthy fats and healthy fats. We want to focus on those healthy fats so that our body's systems are not compromised by being unhealthy.

The great news is that this means you can still enjoy all those desserts just like before! The only difference is the desserts will have a focus on whole foods and healthier fats. Butter can be your friend again, avocado is a good thing, and a wide range of other foods you might be surprised that you can eat. I promise that once you understand the keto diet more in depth, you will be happy to channel your thinking into a low carb high-fat diet. It will be better for your mental acuity as well as that waistline! Yes, despite it being a high-fat diet the keto diet promotes healthy weight loss. This is because of the metabolic state of ketosis you will be trying to achieve through the diet.

Throughout this chapter, I will be introducing you to the ins and outs of the keto diet, and I will also better explain to you why keto recipes are a perfect companion to your intermittent fasting.

What Is Ketosis and How Does it Work?

Carbohydrates are usually the way we supply energy to both our brain and our body's systems. That involves eating a diet that is high in carbohydrates so that you can maintain basic functions and energy levels. Your body breaks the carbs into glucose. But if you recall what I mentioned above, we want our glucose levels to reduce drastically when fasting or doing the keto diet.

The reason for this is because there is another way to provide energy for your body. This alternative method brings its own host of health benefits – the least of which are slimming down your waistline.

You want to bring your body into a metabolic state known as ketosis. With ketosis, you are effectively cutting your body off of its glucose supply and giving it your stored fat to break down.

Sounds a little too much like science class, does it not? But it is important to understand how your body will change when going through ketosis. This way you can prepare for it and make the necessary adjustments.

Let me forewarn you that the metabolic state of ketosis cannot be achieved within a day. It can take anywhere from three days to three weeks for your body to completely switch over to producing energy through ketosis. So, yes, it is a process. But a worthwhile process!

The liver is your king during this process. It is in your liver where your fatty acids are transformed into ketone molecules. This is important because these molecules are what replaces your glucose molecules. So, instead of getting energy from your carbohydrates which end up producing more fat, you will get energy from your fat directly without adding additional weight on your hips. Sounds like a win-win situation to me!

The crazy thing about this method is that it works, and it often surpasses the job that glucose does. No other dietary method can provide fuel to your brain. But ketosis can. This is why it is such a miracle diet. The ketone molecules are able to pass into the brain channel and directly supply your brain with fuel. This means that no part of your body or mind suffers due to the switch in energy production methods.

With your body now relying completely on fat for its fuel, you can see where all that stored fat will disappear as your body processes it for energy. Therefore a record number of people report big weight drops during their first week of ketosis, because all that stored fat is just waiting to be shed.

That is ketosis in a nutshell! It might seem confusing to tell if you are in ketosis yet, but that is where the signs and symptoms come in.

Am I in Ketosis?

Bear in mind that the symptoms of ketosis are not pleasant. In fact, they can even provide some temporary obstacles that you need to combat. And this makes sense. Remember, you are changing the entire way that your body uses and produces energy – there are bound to be some changes that occur because of that.

Remember when I said patience is a virtue. Well, keep that in mind as you take steps toward changing your lifestyle and eating habits. Both intermittent fasting and the keto diet are lifestyle changes. Yes, they can be used temporarily but you will not see the same results, and you will lose out on the health benefits.

So, at the end of the day how do you know if you have achieved the metabolic state of ketosis? Well, it is actually fairly simple. There are some common signs and symptoms that people experience that will help you identify if you are in ketosis or not. Remember, it is not an immediate process and can take up to three weeks before your body is fully in ketosis.

Are you ready for it? Bad breath. Yes, you read that right. And as horrible as it sounds, this is actually a sign you want to look out for. It can indicate that you are in ketosis. It is a very common symptom, and most people report it. It can take the form of a fruity smell or just an overall bad smell.

The compound acetone is at fault for this. It's a main component of the ketone molecules, and it is expelled from the body either by your urine or your breath. Not very sexy, I know. But there are ways to combat this luckily! You can brush your teeth several time throughout the day and make use of sugar-free mints and gums. I say sugar-free because some mints or gums have carbs in them. Remember that you do not want to add unnecessary carbs to your diet!

Of course, one of the main signs is your weight loss. Yes, the long-awaited sign! Both long-term and short-term weight loss are side effects that you will experience while on the keto diet. Bet I just made your day with that bit of news, right? You will see a bigger drop in weight during the first week of keto because all your stored carbs will be used up. This causes the loss of a lot of water weight. Once the big drop is over, your weight loss will be more consistent – as long as you follow the diet.

There are other more invasive ways that you can check to see if you are in ketosis. There are two main tests that people use. The first test is looking for the second compound that makes up your ketone molecules known as beta-hydroxybutyrate (BHB for short). Big word I know. But all you need to know is that if you are in ketosis, this will be present in your body. It works by testing your blood ketone levels (similar to blood sugar levels but the opposite, since they do not rely on glucose).

However, in order to test this way, you need to prick your finger. Not everyone's cup of tea. The tests can also be expensive. While they are reliable, most people still seek other methods to test if they are in ketosis or not.

For example, remember what I said about the bad breath? Well, I also mentioned that the acetone compound is expelled through your urine. There are test strips that you can use to test your acetone levels. It is not as accurate as the blood test above, but you will still be able to tell if you are in nutritional ketosis. The reason these strips are more popular than blood tests is that they are a cheaper alternative.

Okay, so I am about to drop one of the most important ways

to tell if you are in ketosis. Take note of this, because it will be brought up again shortly and everything will start to fall into place for you! While in Ketosis, it has been proven that your levels of hunger decrease. So, ketosis can suppress your appetite. It is a common symptom.

Because our hormones change when we change the way we eat and process food, plus the increase of vegetables and protein that the keto diet demands impacts our regular habits for snacking and consuming food.

Exciting stuff!

There is another symptom I would like to talk about. In fact, it appears as a host of symptoms usually. People have aptly named it the "Keto Flu." Your body will be going through a host of changes during this period, and these changes can have a temporary negative effect on you.

While your body is switching over from glucose to ketone molecules, you might feel sick or even sluggish. The first week or two of the keto diet might not leave you feeling your best. You need to anticipate this so that you are not discouraged when you first start!

A good defense can sometimes be the best offense. So, if you know you are going to start this journey, prepare yourself. Increasing your electrolytes can help you combat the initial onset of feelings you experience when making the switch to ketosis. Supplements never hurt either! If you can add potassium, magnesium, and sodium as supplements to your diet, your body will not experience such a shock. These sluggish feelings are mainly attributed to the over-processed foods that we eat on a daily basis. The keto diet does away with all these food types, and that can shock our systems when we deprive them of the salt and unhealthy carbs that they are used to.

In the long-term, these symptoms will all dissipate, and you will be left feeling better than ever. Like fasting, the keto diet brings with it its own host of health benefits.

Do I Count Calories?

What an awesome question! And the answer is simple, with a little bit of a complicated background.

Essentially counting calories on the keto diet is extremely important. But, the kind of calories you are eating are also important. I bet that is a new concept to you. You can eat 900 calories a day, but if they are not good calories for you, then you still will not benefit from eating them.

The ketogenic diet uses a simple ratio. The ratio can be different and adjusted to meet each person's individual needs, but as with the fasting, there is a core ratio that is used. It consists of calories consumed being 75 percent fat, 20 percent protein, and the remaining 5 percent coming from your carbohydrates. A drastic change if your diet mostly consists of carbs right now.

You still want to maintain a calorie deficit when eating, after all this is still a diet. All that means is that you burn more calories than you eat. As long as you maintain a calorie deficit, then you will lose weight.

In the keto diet, your macronutrients are important when calorie counting. Okay, I know it seems like I just threw another big word at you. Once it all sinks in thought, this information will stay with you. Your macronutrients (macros for short) are simple your protein, fat, and carbohydrates. All this will make sense and come together for you soon, I promise. You just need to keep reading. Highlight if that helps, or even take notes.

This is a big step and a big change, and while things may be confusing for a second, once you have read the guide you will be fully equipped and prepared to start this new journey. I believe in you; you just need to believe in yourself now.

So, Are There Benefits?

Okay, I keep mentioning benefits of the keto diet. So, what are they? Well, I have already highlighted weight loss, but there is more to the keto diet than just weight loss.

In fact, the keto diet earned its beginning as a therapeutic diet for children with epilepsy. Yes, you read right. It has been proven that a keto diet helps reduce and even eliminate the number of seizures and the severity of the seizures that someone suffering from epilepsy will experience.

Some women use the keto diet to help manage their polycystic ovarian syndrome (PCOS). Studies have shown that a high carbohydrate diet negatively affect women with PCOS. These studies have all illustrated that the ketogenic diet improved hormone balance for these women which aided their symptoms of PCOS. There are still more experiments being conducted. However, the preliminary results show great benefits for women with PCOS.

Patients who suffer from memory loss have also found that the keto diet can help improve memory issues. Because it improves your brain's function when your body switches to using ketone molecules.

Acne sufferers, I have some good news for you. Among the

keto diet's growing list of benefits, it has been found to reduce acne. The removal of refined and over processed foods causes our face and bodies to break out less than before. Processed carbohydrates are not good for us or our bodies, yet they exist in a lot of the food that is marketed towards us. Subtracting those unhealthy carbs from our lives means clearer skin in the long run. Remember that there is a direct relationship between our acne and what we put into our bodies.

Both intermittent fasting and keto are good for your heart health. On the keto diet, you have cut out all those unnecessary and unhealthy fats and carbs. And cutting the refined foods from your diet leads to having a higher level of good cholesterol in your system. Your levels of bad cholesterol drastically drop as a result, and this is all good for your heart.

Your overall body function and your health should skyrocket. The keto diet has a positive effect on disorders and diseases and is useful in managing a host of health issues. As with any dietary change, there are some people who are not compatible with the ketogenic diet. If you want to make this change, give your doctor a call. They will be able to guide you on what is beneficial to your health.

Time to Check In

Checking in to make sure you understand the topics is important. This is about you and your health, and I want to ensure that you are accurately equipped to make the change and answer questions other people might have about your lifestyle change.

- The basis of the ketogenic diet is to enter a metabolic state known as ketosis.

- Ketosis is where you no longer produce energy using glucose, but instead your stored fat.

- The keto diet is known as a low carb and high-fat diet.

- While it is high fat, it still promotes eating whole healthy fats.

- Your stored fat is processed in the liver and turned into ketone molecules. These molecules can supply fuel not only to your body but also your brain.

- There are several ways to check if your body is in ketosis. Some involve blood tests, and other symptoms can be as easy to spot as bad breath.

- Keto diets have a host of health benefits. These

benefits can range from helping with epilepsy seizures to promoting good heart health.

- Always consult your doctor before making big lifestyle changes. Some people are just not compatible with the ketogenic diet, and that is okay.

Chapter four will show you how to marry both intermittent fasting and the ketogenic diet. They pair well together, and they give you the best results when used in conjunction with one another. Each diet works well on their own and has great benefits, but when they work together, they become a superb lifestyle change.

Chapter Four: Intermittent Fasting and the Keto Diet

Powerhouse Lifestyle Changes

Finally, the moment I have been itching to get to! In this chapter, I am going to explain to you why your best shot at dieting with intermittent fasting is to pair it with the ketogenic diet.

At this point, you have the basics of both intermittent fasting and the keto diet. You also know why on their own both diets have amazing results for weight loss and a person's overall health status.

The keto diet and intermittent fasting have one important goal in common – to get you into the metabolic state we call ketosis. That is one of the main reasons that they work so well together.

You already know that intermittent fasting requires you to section a window of time where you can eat. By doing this, you are already restricting the amount of food available to you, and your body will begin to look for other outlets to use as energy as your glucose levels drop. This is where your stored fat kicks in.

It happens however that you can negate the progress you make by consuming too many carbs when you finally do eat. This is where the keto diet comes into play. If you maintain the ketogenic diet while you are intermittent fasting, you keep your body in the perfect state of ketosis. You also avoid your body slipping back and forth between using glucose and ketone molecules.

Switching back and forth can be hard on your body. Nobody wants to keep reliving the symptoms you feel when first entering ketosis, so it is a good idea to just stay within good blood ketone levels.

If your ultimate goal is weight loss, then there is no better diet combination than intermittent fasting and keto. The reason lies in how they compliment each other well. If you recall one of the benefits that you get with the keto diet is that it acts as an appetite suppressant. So, in other words, you will not be hungry and constantly snacking.

When you join keto and intermittent fasting, you essentially walk around in fat burning mode all day. With this method, your blood sugar levels should be low – not too low though – and stable. That is why these diets have proven to be so effective for people who are type 2 diabetic or at risk for type 2 diabetes. With a high carb diet you often experience mood swings, cravings and fatigues, those adverse effects are enough to make anyone switch to a low carb high-fat diet.

So, subtract your cravings, suppress your appetite, and suddenly intermittent fasting becomes a whole different ball game. It is a lot easier to manage an intermittent fasting schedule if you pair it with the keto diet. Not only that, but it is the ultimate way to say goodbye to fat safely. You are hitting your fat from two different angles. It does not stand a chance.

Intermittent fasting comes in three states: fed, post-absorptive, and fasted. Your fed state starts right when you begin eating. This state lasts for between three to five hours. This is why a window for eating is best because if you are constantly eating every four hours, your body will never leave the fed state.

Your post-absorptive state can last you between eight to twelve hours after your last meal. Post-absorptive is the state where your body is not processing or digesting a meal. If you are constantly eating, then you will never enter into this stage.

And finally, you have your fasted state. Your fasted state starts twelve hours after the last meal that you ate. So, if you do the 16:8 method, that means that your fasted state will not even start until hour twelve. You will be in the fasted state for four hours before your next meal. The fasted state is where your body naturally burns fat for energy. So, constant eating means that you will never enter into the fasted state, and never experience natural fat burning. With intermittent fasting this state is possible, using the keto diet while intermittent fasting propels your body into a state where it is constantly burning fat.

So, right now you still might be thinking, why do both? Why not just pick one and stick with it?

The answer is so simple it is genius. Intermittent fasting is more difficult to accomplish and stick to on its own. Not only does the keto diet promote healthy eating, but it also suppresses appetite. So intermittent fasting becomes much easier to maintain whilst on the ketogenic diet, and the ketogenic diet gets a big boost from intermittent fasting methods.

Have you ever heard of the term autophagy before? It is a common term that you often hear in conjunction with intermittent fasting. Autophagy is a normal process that your body undergoes during times where food intake is low. It is necessary for your body to go through as it is the process where a cell basically eats itself and recycles what is left in order to make new cells and maintain energy levels.

While you fast and use the keto diet, the process of autophagy increases. In fact, studies have shown that it is a good thing to have high levels of autophagy since low levels can speed up the aging process. So, with higher levels of autophagy, it means that your body is consistently replacing damaged cells and proteins whilst on these two dieting methods.

Let us talk about toning and muscle gain. This can be a hard thing to achieve if you are doing the ketogenic diet on its own. The reason it becomes difficult is that keeping up your exercise performance on the keto diet is not the same as on a high carb diet. Your muscles need glucose for their functions. This is where intermittent fasting steps in to save the day!

Intermittent fasting is actually beneficial to muscle gain and can prevent an extreme loss of muscle mass. When intermittent fasting is done right, you can preserve your muscle mass, and with tweaking your macronutrients on your keto diet to include more protein, you can actually gain muscle mass. Your exercise performance will not be lost at all!

The keto diet improves your mental acuity, gives you an improved attention span, works to prevent cancers, has shown to aid in memory loss patients, suppresses appetite, controls blood sugar levels, and it even aids in controlling and keeping balanced hormones.

Intermittent fasting increases your mental focus, gives you an improved exercise performance, prevents diseases, and increases your overall lifespan. These two powerhouses put together build upon each other's benefits. There are no adverse effects in pairing the two diets, so essentially you have nothing to lose and everything to gain.

Ketogenic studies have proven that the diet can help people with type 2 diabetes and epilepsy. It has also shown that the diet promotes more weight loss than any other diet on the market. And the most amazing results that these studies have proven is the consistent long-term weight loss! A lot of diets you hear about people end up gaining the weight back in a few weeks to a month. With keto, the weight loss continues. As long as you do not overload yourself with high carbs and unhealthy fats, your keto diet should always yield results.

Time to Check In

It is that time again! Just checking in to make sure that the main points stick. There is a lot of information to take in regarding each diet separately, but pairing them together can feel overwhelming. Particularly if you are just starting out on the diet. Take a deep breath. Relax, let us go over the highlights:

- Intermittent fasting has great benefits on its own such

as mental sharpness, weight loss, disease prevention, muscle mass retention, and lifespan longevity.

- The ketogenic diet provides its own great benefits like mental acuity, low blood sugar levels, hormone balance, and reduction of seizures for those that suffer from epilepsy.

- Both forms of fasting and dieting need your body to get into a natural metabolic state known as ketosis.

- Ketosis is the process where your stored body fat is converted in the liver to molecules called ketone molecules.

- Ketone molecules convert into energy that both the brain and body uses.

- When paired, the diets feed off each other in a positive way. They keep your body in a constant fat burning state.

- Keto diets can also reduce your appetite cravings which make intermittent fasting a lot easier to maintain.

That covers the important part of understanding why these two diets go so well together! This guide is mainly focused on women and how they can safely lose weight. In the next chapter, we will explore more about how intermittent fasting can benefit a woman. Since the keto diet has benefits for women who suffer from hormonal imbalances, it is an excellent idea to pair these two diets.

A lot of misconceptions exist regarding woman and intermittent fasting. My goal is to clear these misconceptions up and to be transparent about how, as a woman, you can best utilize intermittent fasting to your advantage. Keep reading! The next chapter is indispensable.

Chapter Five: The Keto Diet, Intermittent Fasting and Women

Is Intermittent Fasting Safe for Me?

There are misconceptions that exist that women cannot intermittent fast. That it is unsafe for them.

Let me stop you in this train of thought right there. A woman can fast safely. In fact, millions of women all over the world fast yearly and benefit from it. But it is important to know what fasting means for you as a woman, and how to best use it to your advantage.

There is no denying that men and women are different. We have different body systems, and they react differently to new changes. That is normal. The key is to find out how to manage the differences. Obviously, one method will not work for every person, regardless if you are male or female. Intermittent fasting is versatile and adaptable to you. That is why it is easy to cater it to ways that fulfill your needs.

In the mainstream news, you might hear a lot of anecdotal evidence of women who experience menstrual changes while fasting. Keep in mind that anecdotal evidence is a far cry from science-based evidence.

You should always consult with your doctor before trying a new lifestyle change. It is recommended that women who already lack their period should not intermittent fast. But what about women who do get their monthly visitor? Should they avoid fasting? Absolutely not. You just need to know how to fast.

Women are sensitive to calorie restriction. The reason is all in our hormones. When there are fewer calories being consumed, the hypothalamus is affected. The hypothalamus is a small part of your brain.

Bear with me, things are going to get a little scientific again. But as women, it is crucial to understand what safe intermittent fasting looks like, and why intermittent fasting affects you differently than it does men.

The effect that a lower amount of calories has on the hypothalamus causes a disruption with the gonadotropin-releasing hormone. GnRH for short. This hormone sounds complicated, but essentially its job is to release two other hormones. The two other hormones are reproductive hormones: a follicle stimulating hormone called FSH for short, and the luteinizing hormone (LH).

All you need to know about these hormones is that they communicate with your ovaries. The disruption of the hypothalamus causes this communication flow to stall. This leads to irregular periods, infertility issues, and in some instances even poor bone health.

But! Do not despair. This does not cancel out intermittent fasting for you as a woman. What it means is that the traditional approach will not work for you. And that is why you are reading this guide because I will walk you through everything you need to know in order to ensure your health is boosted by intermittent fasting and not adversely affected.

So, what does a modified fasting schedule look like? In short, it just means you need to take shorter fasts and have fewer fasting days in your schedule. Also, you need to make use of the ketogenic diet. It will change the entire way that intermittent fasting affects you.

Keep in mind that, despite the negative effects that can be combatted with effectively managing your fasting schedule, intermittent fasting has a host of health benefits for women.

Yes, think about that waistline! When was the last time you looked at your waistline and felt satisfied with it? Well, intermittent fasting can help you attain those waistline goals. Going beyond your waistline, fasting can also greatly reduce your risk for chronic health diseases. These benefits are so worth the lifestyle change. Want more detail on exactly what these health benefits are?

Well, do not worry! I am not skimping on any details here.

Do you know what the leading cause of death is worldwide? Heart health; or in other words a lack of heart health. A study was performed in which 16 men and women with heart trouble took part in. These men and women were also classified as obese. Want to know the results?

Bad heart health is a combination of factors. These factors include high blood pressure, high bad (LDL) cholesterol levels, and high triglyceride concentrations. What a mouthful! Well, in the study that I previously mentioned, it took only eight weeks of intermittent fasting before the participants saw a 6 percent decrease in their high blood pressure. 6 percent! All through intermittent fasting.

But wait! There is more to this. The same study yielded amazing results when it came to cholesterol levels and triglycerides. Bad cholesterol dropped an average of 25 percent, and triglycerides decreased by a staggering 32 percent. Tell me that is not good news for your heart?

More studies are still being done to better understand how intermittent fasting promotes good health and how far the benefits reach.

If you have type 2 diabetes, or perhaps are pre-diabetic, then you should consider using fasting and keto to manage it. There are two things these diets do in order to reduce your risk or eliminate your diabetes. The first is that it lowers your levels of insulin, the second is that it reduces your insulin resistance.

Experts took 100 women who were deemed overweight or obese and put them in a controlled study. Over a period of six months, insulin levels were reduced by 29 percent. This is all through using intermittent fasting. Insulin resistance also dropped by 19 percent in these same women.

I know I have expounded a lot on weight loss. But let me clarify on how it can help you as a woman, or what the weight loss looks like for a woman who chooses to intermittently fast.

In 2018 a wide variety of studies involving intermittent fasting and weight loss were reviewed. It found that between 3-12 months of intermittent fasting an average 15 pounds were lost. Now keep in mind this number is grossly affected by how well you maintain your lifestyle change and how much weight you have to lose in the first place.

The same study reviews indicated that the average reduction in waistline inches was around 3-7 percent over a period of 3-24 weeks.

The natural result of an intermittent fasting lifestyle is that you eat less or less frequently than you normally would. As a woman, you need to still maintain a higher level of food intake than a man. Pairing the keto diet with intermittent fasting would resolve this problem. You can eat larger portions of foods with healthy fat that still meet your calorie requirements for the day. And you can stay in ketosis!

I am going to throw a curveball at you. Intermittent fasting has psychological benefits that extend beyond your mental sharpness. A study was conducted for an extended period, and it concluded with results that indicated that over an eight-week period in which intermittent fasting was used depression decreased in obese and overweight adults. Not only that, but it also improved their binge eating habits and improved their overall body image.

Who does not want to look in the mirror and feel content with what they see? I know I do, and I know you do, too. That is why intermittent fasting can help you get on the right track with body positivity!

The results all lead to intermittent fasting, reducing inflammation in the body as well. This is important because body inflammation leads to several chronic health issues. With this being reduced, it lowers your risk for other health issues.

The bottom line? Yes, intermittent fasting is safe for women, and in fact, has several health benefits that women should take advantage of.

What Kind of Fasting Schedule Do I Need?

Women need a different approach to intermittent fasting than men. Intermittent fasting is already not a one size fits all situation, and its versatility will help you shift and shape a schedule that works for you.

There are a few methods that professionals have already outlined as safe and viable for women. The standard 16:8 method might not work for you, but these others will!

As a woman, one of these methods is going to be the most effective for your goals. Your approach to intermittent fasting should be slightly more laid back than a man's approach. This way you can avoid those adverse effects I mentioned earlier.

The most popular intermittent fasting method for women is the crescendo method. With this, you fast between 12 to 16 hours in a day. The catch is that you only do it for two or three days a week, depending on what suits you best. The days that you choose to fast should be spread out throughout the week. Do not fast back to back days. For example, if you fast on Monday, resume regular eating on Tuesday and fast again on Wednesday. This way you are ensuring that you still eat an adequate amount of food.

The eat-stop-eat is also a good schedule to maintain as a

woman. It is also known as the 24-hour protocol. What this includes is that once or twice a week you do a full twenty-four hour fast. You cannot exceed two times a week with this method. Do not just dive into a full twenty-four fast when you are starting out. Ease into the method. Start with eleven or sixteen hour fast days and work your way up.

The 5:2 diet is another good option. It is different from the other methods because it asks you to restrict calories for two days out of the week. Generally, on intermittent fasting your calories do not need to be counted, but there is an exception for this schedule. This means that for two days a week your goal should be to eat only between 500-600 calories. The other five days of the week you can eat normally. You also need to separate the days of lowered calories with a regular normal eating day.

There is a schedule where you restrict calories every other day. It is called the modified alternate day fasting method. Keep in mind that you need to resume regular eating on your non-fasting days, and the days you fast just keep calories between 500-600. It is a more extreme method of the 5:2 diet, but it still yields results for women without compromising their health.

If you really like the approach of the 16/8 method, you can try it. But be aware that you should not start out at 16 hours of fasting. Gradually work your way up to it. Start with fasting for around 12-14 hours and move up in 15-minute increments when you feel like you are ready. It is important that this method is paired with the keto diet so that you avoid any negative side effects.

Whichever method you choose, you need to make sure it fits into your schedule and life. Maintain healthy eating habits, and you will see results.

Are you ready to get started? Not quite yet, but almost. Getting started is actually really easy.

The odds are that you have already fasted intermittently throughout your life, even if it was not on a consistent basis. Intermittent fasting can be as simple as skipping one meal, whether that is breakfast, lunch, or dinner is up to you.

Choose one of the methods described and give it a go. Try to fit it into your schedule. If you find one is not meant for you, give a different variation a try. You get to pick the hours and meals that best suit you.

Please remember that if you are pregnant, intermittent fasting is not an option for you.

Time to Check In

That was a lot of ground about women and intermittent fasting. I know your head must be swimming with details right now, so let us get back to basics:

- Women can intermittent fast safely. It just needs to be modified from conventional methods.

- There are great health benefits to women who intermittent fast, these include a smaller waistline and lowered risk for type 2 diabetes.

- The crescendo method is the safest and most popular fasting method for women.

- If you are pregnant, you cannot fast intermittently.

The next chapter is going to teach you how to count those macronutrients, and what kind of meals work for intermittent fasting and the keto diet.

Chapter Six: Counting Macronutrients and Meal Plans

How to Count Macronutrients

What a fun topic! Math!

I promise you, though, it becomes simple to understand and is even more practical once you start using it in your daily life.

Counting your macronutrients is important, especially if you are pairing the ketogenic diet with intermittent fasting – which this guide highly recommends that you do for optimal results. Earlier I mentioned that the keto diet works with a ratio for your macronutrients: 75 percent fat, 20 percent protein, and 5 percent carbs.

You need to make sure that you are getting the right number of each macronutrients to keep your body in nutritional ketosis. Your macros will be found in all the foods that you eat, and normally you will see them measured in grams. So, pay attention to the nutritional labels of the foods that you eat. This is the easiest way you can find the macronutrient count. A quick google search will also help you locate the food item that you are unsure of.

Remember, a calorie deficit is still necessary to keep fat burning and weight loss active. That means that if you eat 1800 calories a day you need to burn off 2000 calories. Your macros make up your calorie count.

Your calorie to gram ratio for macros is as follows:

- 9 calories per 1 gram of fat

- 4 calories per 1 gram of carbs

- 4 calories per 1 gram of protein

This might seem a little much right now but bear with me. The keto diet's focus is not just on counting calories like so many other diets out there – but on counting the right kind of calories.

It does not matter if you have a 200-calorie deficit in your diet if all the calories you are eating are from unhealthy fats and refined carbs.

Counting your macros becomes a simple task. In essence, all you do is add up the total grams of protein, fat, and carbs that you eat each day. I am going to give you an example so that it makes plain sense.

Imagine that you have a packet of rice crisps. The rice crisp packet says that one serving size is two crisps. You eat four rice crisps, so you have eaten double the serving size. You need to know what your macros were. Remember, all this information can be found on the nutritional label. Since you ate twice the serving size, you would need to multiply the numbers by two.

So, if two rice crisps had 4g of protein, 3g of fat and 0.5g of carbs you would multiply these numbers by two to get the accurate number of macronutrients that you consumed. Therefore, you would have consumed a total of 8g of protein, 6g of fat, and 1g of carbs.

This method allows you to control how much of each ratio you are eating, and it helps you ensure that you are not overindulging in those carbs. Remember that chart I gave you about how many calories are in each macro? You can easily calculate it here, but we are going to go one step further. First, I want to expand a little more on what your macronutrients are.

Let us start with carbohydrates. These will be found in starches, grains, and foods with high sugar content. If you love breads and sodas, it is time to break up with them because they are loaded with carbs.

This is normally the main way that your body is used to getting energy. Your carbs get broken down into the glucose cells that you use for energy to fuel your bodily systems and functions. But, we want to stop this process from happening.

That is why carbs are so limited on the keto diet because glucose levels need to stay low. Eating a high amount of carbs defeats the purpose of intermittent fasting and the keto diet, and it is not beneficial to your goals. Plus, this is the main reason for all that acne you get.

The largest part of your keto diet is comprised of fats. Fatty diets provide the necessary fat levels our livers need in order to produce ketone molecules. I am not going to flog a dead horse, I am sure you are aware of the process of ketosis by now.

But it is important to note that the fat content is what makes those critical changes to hormone production and our nutrient absorption. Despite it being a high-fat diet, you still want to consume healthy fats. Focus on avocados, butter, oils, and fish high in fat content. Your unhealthy fats will not help you or do you any justice on the keto diet.

Your final macronutrient is the protein. Your body will not function without protein as they are the key component in any function that your body does. Moving your pinky finger? Yes, a protein is behind that. Proteins are essential for all cell signaling, tissue building, immune systems, and hormone and enzyme creation. Getting enough proteins is critical, and you should aim for between twenty to twenty-five percent of your calories to come from proteins. Looking for foods that will meet your protein needs? Try eggs, fish, and tofu!

On to the part you have been waiting for – counting your macros. This part has to be personalized for every person because it varies. Why? Depending on your age, gender, weight, body mass index (BMI), and activity level the amount of calories you need to consume will change.

You need to be able to count your macros correctly, and for this, you need to first know how many calories you need to consume each day. Stay with me, this part can get a little tricky.

There are two components that go into calculating your caloric needs. There are online calculators you can use to do this, but if you prefer to do the math on your own, I will provide a detailed sample here, so you know what to look for.

You need to find out what your resting energy expenditure and your non-resting energy expenditure are (REE and NREE respectively). Your resting energy expenditure are naturally the calories you will burn when your body is at rest – this includes the time you spend sleeping. The crazy thing about our bodies is that we still burn calories even when we are not moving much. Your non-resting energy expenditure are all the calories you burn when you are active.

The total amount of daily calories that you need will be the addition of your REE and NREE. The result is called your total daily energy expenditure, or TDEE for short.

The best way to calculate what this is will be by using the Mifflin-St. Jeor equation. For women it goes as follows:

Calories per day = 10 x weight (kg) + 6.25 x height (cm) − 5 x age (y) − 161.

So, let us say that you are a woman who weighs 60 kgs, has a height of 165 cm, and is 38 years old. Your calculations would look as followed:

Calories per day = 10 x 60kg + 6.25 x 165cm − 5 x 38 − 161 = X

Pretty simple when you visualize it, right?

Okay, there is just one more step to this. The answer from that equation needs to be multiplied by your activity level. This is just based on how active your lifestyle is.

The levels are as follows:

- Sedentary (limited to no exercise) x 1.2

- Lightly active (less than three days a week) x 1.375

- Moderately active (most days of the week) x 1.55

- Very active (every day of the week) x 1.725

- Extra active (exercise two or more times a day) x 1.9

The result from the first equation multiplied by your activity level will provide you with the amount of calories you use every day. The reason this number is so important is because it plays a crucial role in ensuring you meet your calorie deficit for the day in order to lose weight.

The next step in this process is tracking how many of each macronutrient you can eat a day! Because everyone's caloric needs will differ, I am just going to use a base number for the sample. Remember to substitute your own numbers when doing the calculations.

Tracking your macronutrients can be done in any way that is easiest to you. There are apps, journals, notepads, and even websites that you can use to track your macro information. Find a tool that works for you and make use of it. It will become your best friend.

For our macro counting sample, we will be using a 2000 calorie diet and basing it off the sample ratio for the keto diet which is 75 percent fat, 20 percent protein, and 5 percent carbs. Do you remember the calorie per gram breakdown?

Carbohydrates have 4 calories in one gram. So we only need 5 percent of our daily consumption to be from carbs. 5 percent of 2000 calories equals 100 carb calories per day. Now since there are 4 calories in 1 gram, we will divide the 4 by 100. Example:

100calories/4calories per gram = 25 grams of carbs per day.

This is an easy way to keep track of the amount of carbs that you are eating daily. If the nutritional label says you have over 30 grams of carbs in one serving, it is not the meal for you!

Proteins also have 4 calories per gram. And 20 percent of 2000 calories gives us 400 calories of protein per day. So, 400calories/4calories per gram = 100 grams of protein that can be consumed per day.

Healthy fats are supposed to be 75 percent of our diet, and there are 9 calories in 1 gram of fat. 75 percent of a 2000 caloric diet is 1,500 fat calories a day. Your 1500calories/9calories per gram = 166 grams of fat.

It still might seem complicated, but once you put it into practice, it will all fall into place. Keep practicing with counting your macros. Practice makes perfect after all! These numbers are important because you will always be able to refer to them to ensure you are eating the correct amounts of macronutrients a day.

Meal Plans and Why Mean Planning Helps

You did not think I would give you all this information and then leave you to fend for yourself? No!

My goal is to help you with this journey from start to end. And that includes giving you helpful tips and recipes that will help you plan for your keto diet and intermittent fasting schedule.

Depending on your schedule and the kind of personality you have, meal planning might be your best friend. If that is the case then I have some good news for you, I have a host of recipes that you can make, store, and save for another day.

If you are not naturally a meal planner, consider one of the recipes that you can make and eat later, particularly the ones that serve as light snacks. It can be easier to stick to your diet and schedule if you have food already planned ahead or prepped ahead. It also prevents you from falling back into old habits.

Get ready for some homework. You need to make a complete overhaul of your kitchen. What does this look like? Any food in your kitchen that does not follow the nutritional guidelines for the ketogenic diet needs to go. The reason for this is because it makes it substantially easier to cook and eat when you do not have to avoid half of your kitchen.

Meal planning has several benefits. The basics of the benefits include an easier ability to achieve your fitness and diet goals. You tend to eat better meals and spend less money when you meal plan. Who does not like saving money? Meals that are planned out in advance also save you time in the long run. They also help you reduce waste.

Are you ready for some recipes?

Here are some breakfast meal plans to follow:

Egg Muffins the Keto Way

Ingredients:

12 eggs

2 scallions (chopped)

5 ounces of salami or cooked bacon

6 ounces of grated cheese

Salt and pepper to taste

Directions:

- Preheat the oven to 350 degrees F.

- Chop the scallions and salami. Stuff a greased muffin pan with them.

- Mix eggs and seasonings together with the cheese. Combine well and pour egg batter on top of the scallions and salami.

- Bake for 18 minutes until done. These are great to prepare in a big batch ahead of time. You can refrigerate the muffins for up to four days or freeze them to keep them fresher longer.

Devilled Eggs

Ingredients:

4 eggs

1 teaspoon Tabasco

¼ cup mayonnaise

8 pieces of cooked shrimp or salmon

Seasoning to taste

Fresh Dill

Directions:

- Bring water in a medium pot to boil over a medium heat. Place the eggs in water and cover. Boil the eggs for eight to ten minutes to achieve a hard boil.

- Cool the eggs in an ice bath before peeling them. Once cooled and peeled, cut each egg in half and take out the hardened yolk.

- Arrange the egg whites on a separate plate.

- Mix together the mashed egg yolks with Tabasco, mayonnaise, and the seasonings.

- Place this mixture back into the center of the split egg whites. Place a piece of shrimp or the smoked salmon on top of each egg and garnish it with fresh dill.

Italian Breakfast Casserole

Casseroles are a great option for meal planning! They are easy to make in big batches and convenient to store in the freezer for a later date. They are also so versatile, you can do so many different things with them!

Ingredients:

7 ounces cauliflower

2 ounces of butter

8 eggs

12 ounces of Italian sausage

1 cup of heavy whipping cream

5 ounces of grated cheese

Fresh basil

Seasoning to taste

Directions:

- Preheat the oven to 400 degrees F.

- Chop the cauliflower up into tiny florets.

- Melt the butter in the skillet over a medium-high heat

and fry the cauliflower.

- Breaking the sausage up into crumbles fry the pieces until the sausage takes on a golden-brown color.

- Season the cauliflower and sausage mixture to taste.

- Fill a greased baking dish with the cooked mixture.

- Put the basil aside and mix the remaining ingredients together. Season the mixture with salt and pepper. Pour this on top of the sausage and cauliflower mixture. Place the basil on top of this as a garnish.

- Bake the mixture for 35 minutes or until it is golden brown and firm in the middle. Cover the casserole with foil if it is getting too brown before cooking is done. Allow it to finish cooking until set.

Banana Waffles

I promised that you would not have to give up all the things you love when you combine the keto diet and intermittent fasting! Banana waffles are a great keto breakfast that you can enjoy. You could also do breakfast for dinner if you decide to skip on breakfast with your fasting schedule! The other great thing about this recipe is that it is easy to freeze and use as needed! So, you can whip up a big batch and have an easily accessible snack for the next two weeks.

Ingredients:

1 banana (it must be ripe)

4 eggs

¾ of almond flour

¾ coconut milk

1 tablespoon ground psyllium husk powder

Salt to taste

1 teaspoon baking powder

1 teaspoon ground cinnamon

½ teaspoon vanilla extract

Directions:

- Mix all the ingredients together into a batter and let them chill for 20 minutes in the fridge.

- These can be made in a waffle maker or fried in a frying pan, whichever you prefer. Just make sure to fry them in either coconut oil or butter.

- Eat them with whipped coconut cream. Add some fresh berries to add another dimension of taste! There are endless toppings possibilities. Who said you cannot have flavor and keto in the same meal?

Coffee with Cream

Ingredients:

> ¾ cup black coffee brewed the way you like it

> 4 tablespoons heavy whipping cream

Directions:

- Make your coffee the way that you like it. Pour the cream into a small saucepan and heat it gently while stirring.

- Stir until it gets frothy.

- Pour the warm cream into a large cup, add coffee and stir. Serve straight away as is, or with a handful of nuts or a piece of cheese.

Pancakes with Berries and Whipped Cream

Ingredients:

> 4 eggs

> 7 ounces cottage cheese

> 1 tablespoon ground psyllium husk powder

> 2 ounces butter or coconut oil

Toppings:

½ cup fresh raspberries or fresh blueberries or fresh strawberries

1 cup heavy whipping cream

Directions:

- Add the eggs, cottage cheese, and the ground psyllium husk powder into a bowl and then mix it all together. Let this sit for about 5-10 minutes in order to thicken it up.

- Heat up the butter or oil in a skillet that is non-stick and pour in a small amount of batter once it is hot.

- Fry the pancakes on a low to medium heat for about 3 to 4 minutes on each side. Do not make them too big or else they will be hard to flip.

- Add heavy whipping into a separate bowl and whip the cream until soft peaks form. This is how you know it is ready.

- Serve the pancakes with the whipped cream you made and any berries of your choice.

Low Carb Strawberry Smoothie

Ingredients:

14 ounces coconut milk

1 cup fresh strawberries

1 tablespoon lime juice

½ teaspoon vanilla extract

Directions:

- Place all ingredients in a blender and blend until smooth. Using canned coconut milk (drain off the liquid) makes a creamier, more satisfying smoothie. Add lime juice to taste.

Keto Hot Chocolate

Ingredients:

1-ounce unsalted butter

1 tablespoon cocoa powder

1 teaspoon powdered erythritol (optional)

¼ teaspoon vanilla extract

1 cup boiling water

Directions:

- Put the ingredients in an immersion blender.

- Mix them for 15–20 seconds, or until there's a foam on top.

- Pour the hot cocoa carefully into to cups and enjoy.

Remember that if you eat chocolate that it must be dark. White chocolate and milk chocolate are not part of the keto diet.

Frittata with Fresh Spinach

Ingredients:

> 5 ounces diced bacon or chorizo
>
> 2 tablespoons butter, for frying
>
> 8 ounces fresh spinach
>
> 8 eggs
>
> 1 cup heavy whipping cream
>
> 5 ounces grated cheese
>
> Season to taste

Directions:

- Preheat the oven to 350 degrees F.

- Fry the bacon in the butter on a medium-high heat until it is crispy. Add the spinach and stir until it is wilted.

- Remove from the heat and set the pan to the side.

- Whisk together the eggs and cream and pour them into a baking dish (9x9 inches) that is greased, or even into ramekins.

- Put the bacon, spinach, and cheese on top of the eggs and place them in the oven's middle rack.

- Bake for around 25 to 30 minutes or until set in the middle and golden-brown on top.

Classic Bacon and Eggs

Ingredients:

4 eggs

5 ounces bacon, in slices

cherry tomatoes (optional)

fresh parsley (optional)

Directions:

- Fry the bacon in a pan on medium-high heat until crispy.

- Put aside cooked bacon on a plate. Leave the bacon grease in the pan.

- Use this same bacon grease pan to fry the eggs.

- Place the pan over medium heat and crack your eggs into the bacon grease.

- You can cook the eggs any way you like to eat them. Sunnyside up eggs require that you leave the eggs to fry on one side and you cover the pan to make sure they get cooked on top. Eggs that are over easy are flipped over after a few minutes and cooked for another minute.

- Cut the tomatoes in half and fry them at the same time as the eggs.

- Salt and pepper to taste.

Cauliflower Hash Browns

Ingredients:

15 ounces cauliflower

3 eggs

½ yellow onion, grated

1 teaspoon salt

2 pinches pepper

4 ounces butter

Directions:

- Rinse, trim them.

- Rinse and trim the cauliflower. Using a grater, grate the cauliflower finely.

- Place the cauliflower in a bowl with the remaining ingredients and mix it. Set the mixture aside for 5 to 10 minutes.

- Melt a large amount of butter or oil on medium heat in a large skillet.

- Try to cook around 3-4 hash browns at a time, so leave room to expedite the cooking process. Use the oven on a low heat to keep the first batches warm while you cook the others.

- Place scoops of the cauliflower mixture in the frying pan and flatten them out carefully until they measure around 3–4 inches in size

- Fry them for around 4 to 5 minutes on each side. Adjust your heat setting to make sure they don't burn. Remember that patience is key. If you flip the pancakes too quickly, they may fall apart!

Coconut Porridge

Ingredients:

1-ounce butter or coconut oil

1 egg

1 tablespoon coconut flour

1 pinch ground psyllium husk powder

4 tablespoon coconut cream

Salt to taste

Directions:

- Add all the ingredients to a non-stick saucepan. Mix them well and place over a low heat. Stir this mixture constantly until you achieve your desired porridge texture.

- Serve it with either coconut milk or cream. Top your coconut porridge off with a few fresh berries and enjoy it while it is hot!

Scrambled Eggs and Halloumi Cheese

Ingredients:

3 ounces halloumi cheese, diced

4 ounces bacon, diced

2 tablespoon olive oil

2 scallions

4 eggs

½ cup fresh parsley, chopped

½ cup pitted olives

Season to taste

Directions:

- Slice up some halloumi cheese and bacon bits.

- Heat the olive oil on medium-high in a frying pan and fry the halloumi, scallions, and bacon together until they are nicely browned.

- In a bowl, mix together the parsley, eggs, salt, and pepper.

- Place the egg mixture into the frying pan on top of the bacon and cheese bits. Turn the heat to low, add the olives and mix for a couple of minutes.

- Serve with or without a salad.

All these recipes are meant just to get you jump started on breakfast the Keto way! There are so many more recipes you can find, and even more that you can configure yourself. Once you get into the swing of the keto diet, I am confident you will come up with your own tasty recipes!

Honestly, there are hundreds of amazing breakfast keto recipes out there that you can pair with your fasting schedule. You do not have to restrict yourself at all!

Did someone say Lunch? I know that for those who skip breakfast, lunch will, in turn, become your most important meal of the day. But how do you plan so that you do not binge or eat those unhealthy fats? Simple! Use some of these recipes to get started on lunch ideas on keto. Who knows where they might take you?

Tuna Cheese Melt

If you are giving me the side eye right now, take it back. I will not steer you in the wrong direction. I know you need bread in order to make a tuna cheese melt. Or do you? I am so excited to introduce to you a great keto alternative to bread that you can easily make yourself and freeze at home for use at a later date! It is called oopsie bread!

Oopsie Bread Ingredients (yields 6-8 pieces):

3 eggs

4 ounces of cream cheese

Salt to taste

½ tablespoon ground psyllium husk powder

½ teaspoon baking powder

Directions:

- Preheat the oven to 300 degrees F.

- You need to separate the egg yolks from the egg whites. Take the egg whites, add salt to taste, and whip them until they are stiff. When you turn the bowl upside down that egg white should remain still.

- Cream together the egg yolks and cream cheese. The psyllium husk powder and baking powder are optional. They just make it have a bread-like consistency. If you add them, fold them into the egg yolk mixture.

- Fold the egg whites into the egg yolk mixture.

- Scoop 8 pieces onto a baking tray that is lined with parchment paper and bake them for 25 minutes. Or until they appear golden.

Tuna Fish Salad Ingredients:

1 cup of mayonnaise or sour cream

4 stalks of celery

½ cup of chopped dill pickles

1 teaspoon lemon juice

1 minced garlic clove

Salt and pepper to taste

8 ounces of tune in olive oil

Grated cheese

Directions:

- Preheat the oven to 350 degrees F.

- Mix together all the salad ingredients.

- Spread the tuna mix over your oopsie bread that has been cooked. The bread should be on a baking sheet that has been lined with parchment paper. Add some more cheese on top of the tuna mixture.

- Bake the melt in the oven until the cheese turns golden. This should take 15 minutes.

Tuna Salad with Capers

A nice refreshing salad can make a great meal on a hot day. Tuna salads are healthy and filling.

Ingredients:

4 ounces tuna in olive oil

½ cup mayonnaise

2 tablespoons fresh cream

1 tablespoon capers

½ leek

½ teaspoon chili flakes

Season to taste

Directions:

- Drain the oil from the tuna and mix all the ingredients together. Remember to finely chop the leek, so it melds with the rest of the salad.

- Season the tuna mixture to taste with salt and pepper. This dish can be served alongside boiled eggs or oopsie bread (refer to recipe above).

Keto Quesadillas

Quesadillas can be prepped ahead of time for the same day, but they do not do well frozen. These are a great option if you are entertaining a group and want to be able to eat with them! There are several parts to making these quesadillas!

Low-carb Tortillas –

Ingredients:

2 eggs

2 egg whites

6 ounces cream cheese

1½ teaspoon ground psyllium husk powder

1 tablespoon coconut flour

½ teaspoon salt

Directions:

- Preheat the oven to 400 degrees F.

- Beat the eggs together until they appear fluffy. Add the cream cheese and continue to whisk the mixture until the batter seems smooth and has no lumps.

- Mix together the salt, psyllium husk powder, and coconut flour in a medium bowl. Make sure they are mixed well. Sift the flour mixture into the egg batter while mixing continuously. When fully combined, let the batter rest. Be careful not to over mix this batter. It should have a thick pancake-like consistency. If it does not seem to be thick enough after it rests, be patient and add some more psyllium husk powder. Do this gradually so that you do not add to much husk powder into the mixture.

- Place some parchment paper on a baking sheet. Using a spatula spread the batter over the parchment paper. If you want your tortillas to be round, you can fry them in a frying pan just as you do for pancakes. This all depends on your preference.

- Bake the tortillas on the top rack for around 6 minutes. You will know that the tortilla is done because the edges will begin to turn brown Watch the oven carefully because they can burn on the bottom quickly if you do not keep a close eye on them.

- Cut the main tortilla into 6 smaller tortilla pieces in order to make the quesadillas.

Filling –

Ingredients:

5 ounces grated Mexican cheese or hard cheese

1-ounce arugula lettuce

Directions:

- For the quesadillas, heat a non-stick skillet. If you want to fry the quesadilla, you need to add a little bit of oil to the skillet. Place the tortilla in the frying pan and sprinkle it with some cheese, the greens, and add some more cheese on top of the greens. Top this with another tortilla.

- Fry each quesadilla for about one minute on each side. You will know that it is done when the cheese melts.

Chicken Curry Pie

This recipe is a great one to make ahead and freeze! It keeps well and tastes even better the day after it is made! You can save them for a rainy day or stock up for meals for the month ahead. Whatever you decide to do, this chicken curry pie is a must make!

Pie Crust –

Ingredients:

¾ cup of almond flour

4 tablespoons sesame seeds

4 tablespoons coconut flour

1 tablespoon ground psyllium husk powder

1 teaspoon baking powder

Salt to taste

3 tablespoons olive oil

1 egg

4 tablespoons water

Filling –

Ingredients:

10 ounces cooked chicken

1 cup mayonnaise

3 eggs

½ green bell pepper, finely chopped

1 teaspoon curry powder

½ teaspoon paprika powder

½ teaspoon onion powder

¼ teaspoon ground black pepper

½ cup cream cheese

1¼ cups shredded cheese

Directions:

- Preheat the oven to 350 degrees F.

- Using a food processor, place all the ingredients for the pie crust into one and process them all together for a few minutes, just long enough until the dough forms into a ball. You can also mix the dough using a fork if you prefer to do it that way or if you are missing a food processor in your kitchen.

- Place a piece of parchment paper onto a pan that is no larger than 10 inches around. Grease the bottom and sides of the dish.

- The dough must be spread into the pan. Use an oiled spatula or your oil-coated fingers to do this. The crust must bake for 12 to 15 minutes before you add any filling.

- Combine the other filling ingredients, and fill the baked pie crust. Bake this for an additional 35 to 40 minutes. Or until the pie color has turned a golden-brown.

- Let the pie cool and then serve it with a salad and light dressing.

Salmon Pie

Like the chicken pie, the salmon pie is great for meal planning since you can store in the fridge or the freezer! Once this is done, you can just relax for the rest of the week! Meal planning really can be simple.

Pie Crust –

Ingredients:

   ¾ cup of almond flour

   4 tablespoons sesame seeds

   4 tablespoons coconut flour

1 tablespoon ground psyllium husk powder

1 teaspoon baking powder

Salt to taste

3 tablespoons olive oil

1 egg

4 tablespoons water

Filling –

Ingredients:

8 ounces smoked salmon

1 cup mayonnaise

3 eggs

2 tablespoons fresh dill, finely chopped

½ teaspoon onion powder

¼ teaspoon ground black pepper

4¼ ounces cream cheese

1¼ cups shredded cheese

Directions:

- Preheat the oven to 350 degrees F.

- Place the dough ingredients into a food processor that is meant to mix pastry. Mix this until the mixture forms a ball. If you don't have a food processor, another way to mix the dough is with a fork.

- Fit some parchment paper into a 10-inch pan.

- Coat your fingers or a spatula in oil, and gently press the dough into the springform pan. Bake the crust for 10 to 15 minutes, or until it is lightly browned.

- Keeping the salmon aside, combine the other ingredients for the filling and pour that in with the pie crust. Add the salmon to this mixture now and bake it for 35 minutes, or until the pie is golden-brown.

- Let the pie cool for a few minutes before serving or storing it.

Keto Cabbage Stir Fry

Ingredients:

25 oz. green cabbage

5⅓ oz. butter

20 oz. ground beef

1 tsp salt

1 tsp onion powder

¼ tsp pepper

1 tbsp white wine vinegar

1 tbsp tomato paste

2 garlic cloves, finely chopped

3 oz. leeks, thinly sliced

½ cup fresh basil

1 cup mayonnaise or sour cream, for serving

Directions:

- Shred the green cabbage finely with either a sharp knife or in a food processor.

- Fry the cabbage in the butter. Olive oil can be used as a substitute. Fry it in a large frying pan or a wok on medium heat for 10 minutes, or until it is softened.

- Add the vinegar, onion powder, salt, and pepper. Continue to stir it and fry for 2 to 3 minutes, or until well mixed. Move the sautéed cabbage to a bowl.

- Heat the rest of the butter or olive oil in the same pan. Add the garlic and leeks, and sauté them for a minute until they get a little soft.

- Add the meat, and continue stirring until it is cooked

through. Sauté until most of the liquid has gone and your meat is brown.

- Mix it well while adding tomato paste. Turn the heat down slightly and add the saved cabbage and fresh basil. Stir until it is cooked through.

- Adjust the seasoning as needed and serve with a dollop of sour cream or mayonnaise.

This is an absolutely yummy stir fry! It also freezes well, so when you are in the mood, double it up and save the other half for a rainy day!

Simple Keto Pizza

Ingredients:

Crust -

4 eggs

6 oz. shredded cheese, preferably mozzarella or provolone

Topping:

3 tbsp tomato paste

1 tsp dried oregano

5 oz. shredded cheese

1½ oz. pepperoni

olives (optional)

Directions:

- Preheat the oven to 400 degrees F.

- Start with the crust. Crack eggs into a bowl and add the shredded cheese. Stir it well to combine.

- Using a spatula, spread the cheese and egg batter onto a baking sheet lined with parchment paper. Make two round circles or just make one large rectangular pizza, whichever you prefer. Bake the crust in the oven for 15 minutes until the pizza turns golden. Remove the crust from the oven and let it cool for a minute or two.

- Increase the oven temperature to 450°F.

- Spread the tomato paste over the crust and sprinkle oregano on top. Top this with cheese and add the pepperoni and olives on top.

- Bake the pizza for another 5-10 minutes or until the pizza has turned a golden-brown color. You can serve with a green salad on the side.

Keto Cheeseburger

Ingredients:

25 oz. ground beef

7 oz. shredded cheese

2 tsp garlic powder

2 tsp onion powder

2 tsp paprika powder

2 tbsp fresh oregano, finely chopped

2 oz. butter, for frying

Salsa

2 tomatoes

2 scallions

1 avocado

1 tbsp olive oil

salt

fresh cilantro, to taste

Toppings

¾ cup mayonnaise

5 oz. cooked bacon

4 tbsp Dijon mustard

½ cup sliced dill pickles

5 oz. lettuce

¼ cup pickled jalapeños

Directions:

- Chop the salsa ingredients together and stir them together in a small bowl. Set the mixture aside.

- Pour in seasoning and half of the cheese into the ground beef.

- Shape four burgers from the mixture and fry them in a pan. You can also grill them. Add the remaining cheese on top at the end of cooking.

- Serve on top lettuce with pickle and mustard. Don't forget to add the homemade salsa.

Keto BLT and Cloud Bread

Cloud Bread –

Ingredients:

3 eggs

4¼ ounces cream cheese

1 pinch salt

½ tablespoon ground psyllium husk powder

½ teaspoon baking powder

Toppings:

5 tablespoons mayonnaise

5 ounces bacon

2 ounces lettuce

1 tomato, thinly sliced

fresh basil (optional)

Directions:

- Preheat oven to 300 degrees F.

- Separate the eggs and place the egg whites into a separate bowl than the egg yolks.

- Whip the egg whites together with salt until very stiff. Preferably using a handheld electric mixer. To make sure it is stiff, the bowl should be turned over, and the egg whites should not move.

- Add the cream cheese to the egg yolks and mix these together well. If you want it to be more bread-like, you can add in some baking powder and psyllium seed husk.

- Carefully fold the egg whites into the egg yolk mixture

while trying to keep the air in the egg whites.

- Place 8 cloud bread pieces on a baking tray lined with parchment paper.

- -Bake in the middle rack of the oven for around 25 minutes, until they turn golden brown.

- Building the BLT

- Fry the bacon in a skillet on medium-high heat until crispy.

- The cloud bread pieces get placed top side down.

- Spread 1 to 2 tablespoon of mayonnaise on each slice.

- Place lettuce, tomato, finely chopped fresh basil, and fried bacon in layers between the bread halves. Serve immediately.

From this recipe, you can make quite a few batches of cloud bread at a time and store them! That way you have it on hand when you need them. You can store cloud bread in the fridge for 2-3 days, or in the freezer for up to three months.

Goat Cheese Salad and Balsamic Butter

Ingredients:

10 ounces goat cheese

¼ cup pumpkin seeds

2 ounces butter

1 tablespoon balsamic vinegar

3 ounces baby spinach

Directions:

- Preheat the oven to 400 degrees F.

- Place the slices of goat cheese on a greased baking dish and bake them in the oven for around 10 minutes.

- Toast some pumpkin seeds in a dry frying pan over a moderately high temperature until they get some color and start to pop.

- Once they start to pop, lower the heat and add butter. Let it simmer until it turns a golden-brown color, and a pleasant nutty scent emits from the pan. Add some balsamic vinegar and let it boil for a few more minutes. Turn off and remove from the heat.

- Spread out some baby spinach on a plate. Place the

cheese on top and add the balsamic butter.

Mayonnaise

Homemade mayonnaise is so much better for you than what you can buy in the store. It is also usually tastier, too. Try your hand at this keto friendly recipe:

Ingredients:

1 egg yolk

1 tablespoon Dijon mustard

1 cup avocado oil

2 teaspoons white wine vinegar

Directions:

- Make sure you are using egg and mustard that is at room temperature.

- Mix the egg and mustard together in a blender and add the oil slowly in a thin stream. The mayonnaise should begin to thicken as you do this. Continue to mix well until all the oil has been added and the mayonnaise has set in a firm consistency.

- Add some vinegar or lemon juice to the mayonnaise mixture. Stir it some more and season with salt and pepper. Taste your mayonnaise, and adjust the seasoning according to your preference. Add more vinegar or lemon juice if needed.

- Set the mayonnaise in the fridge before serving to allow it to rest; this lets the flavor develop and gives the mayonnaise time to thicken.

Dinner recipes are particularly important. Depending on your fasting schedule, dinner might be the biggest meal you have for the day. This is why meal prep can be important if you have a busy schedule. This way you ensure that you have a hearty meal that is still within the keto limitations to eat. Keep on reading for some tasty dinner recipes!

Keto Pesto Chicken Casserole

Ingredients:

25 ounces boneless chicken breasts

Butter for frying

3 ounces red pesto

1¼ cups heavy whipping cream

3 ounces pitted olives

5 ounces feta cheese, diced

1 garlic clove, finely chopped

Season to taste

Directions:

- Preheat the oven to 400 degrees F.

- Cut the chicken breasts into bite-sized pieces. Season them with salt and pepper to taste.

- Add the butter to a large skillet and fry the chicken in batches on a medium-high heat until they are golden-brown.

- Mix the pesto and heavy cream together in a small bowl.

- Mix the fried chicken pieces in a baking dish together with the olives, feta cheese, and garlic. Add the pesto to this chicken mixture.

- Bake in the oven for 20 to 30 minutes, until the dish gets bubbly and light brown around the edges.

Keto Tex-Mex Casserole

Ingredients:

25 ounces ground beef

2 tablespoons butter

3 tablespoons Tex-Mex seasoning

7 ounces crushed tomatoes

2 ounces pickled jalapeños

7 ounces shredded cheese

To Serve:

1 cup sour cream

1 scallion, finely chopped

5 ounces leafy greens

1 cup guacamole (optional)

Directions:

- Preheat the oven to 400 degrees F.

- Fry the ground beef in the butter on medium-high heat, until it is cooked through and no longer pink.

- Add some Tex-Mex seasoning and crushed tomatoes. Stir and let simmer for 5 minutes. Taste to see if needs additional salt and pepper.

- Place the ground beef mixture into a greased baking dish (about 9" round). Top it with jalapeños and cheese.

- Bake it on the upper rack in the oven for 15 to 20 minutes, or until golden-brown on top.

- Finely chop the scallion and mix it with the sour cream in a separate bowl.

- The casserole must be served warm with only a dollop of the crème Fraiche or sour cream on top. Some guacamole, and a leafy green salad.

Keto Zucchini Pizza Boats

Ingredients:

1 medium-sized zucchini

2 garlic cloves

4 tablespoons olive oil

2 cups baby spinach

Season to taste

2 tablespoons unsweetened marinara sauce

8 ounces goat cheese

Directions:

- Preheat oven to 375 degrees F.

- Slice the zucchini in half and use a spoon to scrape out the seeds. Reserve the seeds. Preheat oven to 375°F.

- Slice the zucchini in half and use a spoon to scrape out

the seeds. Reserve the seeds and put them aside. Place the zucchini shells on a baking sheet.

- Peel the garlic cloves and thinly slice them with a knife. Using half of the olive oil, fry the garlic in a skillet that is over a medium heat until it is nicely browned. Add the baby spinach and zucchini seeds. Season with salt and ground black pepper to taste.

- The marinara needs to be spread to cover the bottom of the zucchini boats. Stuff the boats with the fried baby spinach and the garlic. Sprinkle goat cheese on top of the boat stuffing.

- Bake for around 20 to 25 minutes or until the zucchini is tender and the cheese has turned a golden color.

- With the remaining half of the olive oil, drizzle this over the cooked zucchini boats. You can add additional season to taste before serving.

Keto Lasagna

This lasagna recipe is by far one of the most challenging recipes in this guide. But I promise you the fruit is so worth the labor! Plus, this is an awesome option for meal prep. The lasagna keeps well in the fridge or freezer and can be served as a hearty meal any night of the week!

Filling -

Ingredients:

2 tablespoons olive oil

1 yellow onion

1 garlic clove

20 ounces ground beef

3 tablespoons tomato paste

½ tablespoon dried basil

1 teaspoon salt

¼ teaspoon ground black pepper

½ cup water

Keto pasta -

Ingredients:

8 eggs

10 ounces cream cheese

1 teaspoon salt

5 tablespoons ground psyllium husk powder

Cheese topping –

Ingredients:

2 cups sour cream

5 ounces grated cheddar cheese

2 ounces grated parmesan cheese

½ teaspoon salt

¼ teaspoon ground black pepper

½ cup fresh parsley, finely chopped

Directions:

- Start with the ground beef mixture. You can prepare this a day or two before you use it for added flavor.

- Peel and finely chop the onion and the garlic. Fry them in olive oil until they are soft. Add the ground beef to the onion and garlic and cook until golden. Add the tomato paste and remaining spices.

- Stir the mixture thoroughly and add some water. Bring it to a boil, turn the heat down, and let it simmer for at least 15 minutes, or until most of the water has evaporated. The lasagna sheets used don't soak up as much liquid as regular ones, so the mixture should be quite dry.

- While that is happening make the lasagna sheets according to the instructions that follow below.

- Preheat the oven to 400 degrees F. Mix the shredded cheese with sour cream and the Parmesan cheese. Reserve one or two tablespoons of the cheese aside for the topping. Add salt and pepper for taste and stir in the parsley.

- Place the lasagna sheets and pasta sauce in layers in a greased baking dish.

- Spread the cream mixture and the reserved Parmesan cheese on top.

- Bake the lasagna in the oven for around 30 minutes or until the lasagna has a nicely browned surface. Serve with a green salad and a light dressing.

Lasagna sheets:

- Preheat the oven to 300 degrees F.

- Add the eggs, cream cheese, and the salt to a mixing bowl and blend into a smooth batter. Continue to whisk this while adding in the ground psyllium husk powder, just a little bit at a time. Let it sit for a few minutes to rest.

- Using a spatula, spread the batter onto a baking sheet that is lined with parchment paper. Place more parchment paper on top and flatten it with a rolling pin until the mixture is at least 13" x 18". You can also divide it into two separate batches and use a different baking sheet for even thinner pasta.

- Let the pieces of parchment paper stay in place. Bake the pasta for about 10 to 12 minutes. Let it cool and remove the paper. Slice into sheets that fit your baking dish.

Slow Cooker Keto Pork Roast

Ingredients:

30 ounces pork shoulder or pork roast

½ tablespoon salt

1 bay leaf

5 black peppercorns

2½ cups water

2 teaspoon dried thyme

2 garlic cloves

1½ ounces fresh ginger

1 tablespoon olive oil or coconut oil

1 tablespoon paprika

½ teaspoon ground black pepper

Creamy gravy:

1½ cups heavy whipping cream

The juices from the roast

Directions:

- Preheat the oven to a low heat of 200 degrees F.

- Season the meat with salt and place it in a deep baking dish.

- Add water to cover 1/3 of the meat. Add a bay leaf, peppercorns, and thyme for more seasoning. Place the baking bowl in the oven for 7 to 8 hours and cover it with aluminum foil.

- If you are using a slow cooker for this, do the same process as in step 2, only add 1 cup of water. Cook it for 8 hours on low or for 4 hours on high setting.

- Take the meat out of the baking dish, and reserve the pan juices in a separate pan to make gravy.

- Turn the oven up to 450 degrees F.

- Finely chop or press the garlic and ginger into a small bowl. Add the oil, herbs, and pepper and stir well to combine.

- Rub the meat with the garlic and herb mixture.

- Return the meat to the baking dish, and roast it for about 10 to 15 minutes, or until it looks golden-brown.

- Cut the meat into thin slices to serve it with the creamy gravy.

Gravy:

- Strain the reserved pan juices to get rid of any solid pieces from the liquid. Boil and reduce the pan juices to about half the original volume. This should be about 1 cup.

- Pour the reduction into a pot with the whipping cream. Bring this to a boil. Reduce the heat and let it simmer for about 20 minutes or to your preferred consistency for a creamy gravy.

Fried Eggs with Kale and Pork

Ingredients:

½ pound kale

3 ounces butter

6 ounces smoked pork belly or bacon

¼ cup frozen cranberries

1-ounce pecans or walnuts

4 eggs

Season to taste

Directions:

- Cut and chop the kale into large squares. You can use pre-washed baby kale as a shortcut if you want. Melt two-thirds of the butter in a frying pan, and fry the kale on high heat until it is slightly browned around its edges.

- Remove the kale from the frying pan and put it aside. Sear the pork belly in the same frying pan until it is crispy.

- Turn the heat down. Put the sautéed kale back in the pan and add the cranberries and nuts. Stir this mixture until it is warmed through. Put it into a bowl on the side.

- Turn up the heat again, and fry the eggs in the remaining amount of the butter. Add salt and pepper to taste. Serve the eggs and greens immediately.

Cauliflower Soup with Pancetta

Ingredients:

4 cups chicken broth or vegetable stock

15 ounces cauliflower

7 ounces cream cheese

1 tablespoon Dijon mustard

4 ounces butter

Season to taste

7 ounces pancetta or bacon, diced

1 tablespoon butter, for frying

1 teaspoon paprika powder or smoked chili powder

3 ounces pecans

Directions:

- Trim the cauliflower and cut it into smaller floret heads. The smaller the florets are, the quicker the soup will be ready.

- Put aside a handful of the fresh cauliflower and chop into small 1/4 inch bits.

- Sauté the finely chopped cauliflower and pancetta in

butter until it is crispy. Add some nuts and the paprika powder at the end. Set aside the mixture for serving.

- Boil the cauliflower florets in the stock until they are soft. Add the cream cheese, mustard, and butter.

- Stir the soup well, using an immersion blender, to get to the desired consistency. The creamier the soup will become the longer you blend. Salt and pepper the soup to taste.

- Serve soup in bowls, and top it with the fried pancetta mixture.

Meatloaf Wrapped in Bacon

Ingredients:

2 tbsp butter

1 yellow onion, finely chopped

25 oz. ground beef or ground lamb/pork

½ cup heavy whipping cream

½ cup shredded cheese

1 egg

1 tbsp dried oregano or dried basil

1 tsp salt

½ tsp ground black pepper

7 oz. sliced bacon

1¼ cups heavy whipping cream, for the gravy

Directions:

- Preheat the oven to 400 degrees F.

- Fry the onion until it is soft but not overly browned.

- Mix the ground meat in a bowl with all the other ingredients, minus the bacon. Mix it well, but avoid overworking it as you do not want the mixture to become dense.

- Form the meat into a loaf shape and place it in a baking dish. Wrap the loaf completely in the bacon.

- Bake the loaf in the middle rack of the oven for about 45 minutes. If you notice that the bacon begins to overcook before the meat is done, cover it with some aluminum foil and lower the heat since you do not want burnt bacon.

- Save all the juices that have accumulated in the baking dish from the meat and bacon, and use to make the gravy. Mix these juices and the cream in a smaller saucepan for the gravy.

- Bring to a boil and lower the heat and let it simmer for 10 to 15 minutes until it has the right consistency and is not lumpy.

- Serve the meatloaf with freshly boiled broccoli or some cauliflower with butter, salt, and pepper.

Keto Salmon with Broccoli Mash

Ingredients:

Salmon burgers -

1½ lbs. salmon

1 egg

½ yellow onion

1 tsp salt

½ tsp pepper

2 oz. butter, for frying

Green mash

1 lb. broccoli

5 oz. butter

2 oz. grated parmesan cheese

salt and pepper to taste

Lemon butter

    4 oz. butter at room temperature

    2 tablespoons lemon juice

    salt and pepper to taste

Directions:

- Preheat the oven to 220 degrees F. Cut the fish into smaller pieces and place them along with the rest of the ingredients for the burger into a food processor.

- Blend it for 30 to 45 seconds until you have a rough mixture. Don't mix it too thoroughly as you do not want tough burgers.

- Shape 6 to 8 burgers and fry them for 4 to 5 minutes on each side on a medium heat in a generous amount of butter. Or even oil if you prefer. Keep them warm in the oven.

- Trim the broccoli and cut it into smaller florets. You can use the stems as well, just peel them and chop it into small pieces.

- Bring a pot of salted water to a boil and add the broccoli to this. Cook it for a few minutes until it is soft, but not until all the texture is gone. Drain and discard the water used for boiling.

- Use an immersion blender or even a food processor to mix the broccoli with the butter and the parmesan cheese. Season the broccoli mash to taste with salt and pepper.

- Make the lemon butter by mixing room temperature butter with lemon juice, salt and pepper into a small bowl using electric beaters. You can also do this by hand with a whisk.

- Serve the warm burgers with a side of green broccoli mash and a melting dollop of fresh lemon butter on top of the burger.

Oven Baked Sausage and Vegetables

Ingredients:

1 oz. butter, for greasing the baking dish

1 small zucchini

2 yellow onions

3 garlic cloves

5⅓ oz. cherry tomatoes

7 oz. fresh mozzarella cheese

½ tsp sea salt

¼ tsp ground black pepper

1 tbsp dried basil or dried thyme

¼ cup olive oil

1 lb. sausages in links, in links

For serving:

1/2 cup mayonnaise

Directions:

- Preheat the oven to 400 degrees F.

- Using butter, grease a baking dish.

- Chop the zucchini into bite-sized pieced. Peel and chop the onion, and you can either slice or dice the garlic.

- Mix the zucchini, garlic, onions, and tomatoes in the oven proof baking dish. Slice the cheese into cubes that are 1-inch thick and place them amongst the vegetables. Then season the mixture to taste with salt, pepper, and basil.

- Take the olive oil and lightly drizzle it over the vegetable mix. Place your sausage links on top of this.

- Bake the dish for at least 40 minutes. This means the

sausages will be cooked through and your onions should be a nice caramelized brown.

- If you want, you can serve it with a spoon of mayonnaise.

Zucchini Fettuccine with Beef

Ingredients:

15 oz. ground beef

3 tbsp butter

1 yellow onion

8 oz. mushrooms

1 tbsp dried thyme

½ tsp salt

1 pinch ground black pepper

8 oz. blue cheese

1½ cups sour cream

Zucchini fettuccine:

2 zucchinis

1 oz. olive oil or butter

salt and pepper

Directions:

- Peel the onion and chop it finely.

- Melt the butter in a pot over a medium heat, and sauté the onion until the onions are softened and transparent.

- Add the ground beef and fry this for a few more minutes with the onion until it is browned and cooked through.

- Slice or dice the mushrooms and add to the ground beef. Sauté the mushrooms with the beef mixture for a few minutes more, or until lightly brown.

- Season with thyme, salt, and pepper. Crumble the cheese over the hot mixture. Stir it well.

- Add the sour cream and bring the mixture to a light boil. Lower the heat to a medium-low setting and let it simmer for 10 minutes.

Zucchini fettuccine:

- Calculate about one medium-sized zucchini per person. Slice the zucchini lengthwise in half.

- Scoop out the seeds with a spoon and slice the halves

super thinly, lengthwise (julienne) with a potato peeler, or you can use a spiralizer to make zoodles (zucchini noodles.)

- Toss the zucchini in some hot sauce of your choice and serve it immediately.

- If you are not going to be serving your zucchini with a hot sauce, then boil half a gallon of salted water in a large pot and parboil the zucchini slices for a minute. This makes them easier to eat

- Drain the water from the pot and add some olive oil or a knob of butter. Salt and pepper to taste and stir the zoodles.

Keto Avocado Quiche

Ingredients:

Pie crust -

¾ cup almond flour

4 tbsp sesame seeds

4 tbsp coconut flour

1 tbsp ground psyllium husk powder

1 tsp baking powder

1 pinch salt

3 tbsp olive oil or coconut oil

1 egg

4 tbsp water

Filling:

2 ripe avocados

1 cup mayonnaise

3 eggs

2 tbsp fresh cilantro, finely chopped

1 red chili pepper, finely chopped

½ tsp onion powder

¼ tsp salt

½ cup cream cheese

1¼ cups shredded cheese

Directions:

- Preheat the oven to 350° F. Mix all the ingredients together for the pie dough in a food processor until the dough forms into a ball. This takes a few minutes usually. Use your hands or a fork in the absence of a food processor to knead the dough.

- Place a piece of parchment paper to the pan, no larger than 12 inches around. The springform pan makes it easier to take the pie out when it is done. Grease the pan and the parchment paper.

- Using an oiled spatula or oil coated fingers, spread the dough into the pan. Bake the crust for 10 to 15 minutes.

- Split the avocado in half. Remove the peel and put it in, and dice the avocado.

- Take the seeds out of the chili and chop the chili very finely. Combine the avocado and the chili in a bowl and mix them together with the other ingredients.

- Pour the mixture into the pie crust and bake it for 35 minutes or until it is a light golden brown. Let it cool for a few minutes and serve it with a green salad

These recipes should all give you a great head start on your way to cooking for keto fasting! Remember that there are a ton of benefits not just from fasting but from the keto diet as well.

Chapter Seven: Thirty Day Action Plan

Putting Theory into Practice

So, by now you are well equipped with the knowledge about what makes both intermittent fasting and the keto diet work so well together! I have exhausted the benefits, counting calories and why it is important for women to take a more relaxed approach to intermittent fasting than men. But what does putting that plan into action look like? What does your plan even look like in the first place?

It is important that your plan of action is established and easy for you to follow, so in this chapter, we are going to focus on setting goals for your first month of fasting on keto! Excited? You should be! This is where all your learning comes to fruit.

You need a weekly goal. Everyone's weight loss journey is going to be different but if you start with a weekly goal then you will be able to lose weight safely, and you can hold yourself accountable for the goals.

Losing two pounds a week is a safe, manageable goal to set for yourself. This might seem like chump change yet but imagine that there are a standard four weeks in one month. That means that in thirty days you stand to lose a total of eight pounds.

Focus on your plan in weekly goals. Here is what it could look like:

Week One – Weigh yourself and set a reasonable expectation for the amount of weight you want to lose. Remember that two pounds is a safe average, but if your goal's focus on half a pound or one pound, that is okay too. Now that you have weight goals in mind, the next step is crucial.

You need to find out what fasting method works best for you. Try the method out for a week to see if it works for you. I advise that you try the Crescendo method first as this is the most popular amongst women and the safest way to intermittent fast. Set a schedule that works for your day and week. Tailor it to your lifestyle.

Clean out your kitchen. This includes your cupboards, fridge, and the secret stash you have hidden that only you know about. Yes, all of it. The keto diet focuses on whole healthy foods and fats. You need to get rid of all the refined carbs and processed foods. Focus on meal planning, I promise it will help you. By clearing out the kitchen, you are lessening possible temptation. A change can be hard, do not make it harder on yourself by keeping old crutches around. Clear out the temptations and start out fresh.

Meal plan! Decide ahead of time what meals you are going to eat this week. Make them purposeful and ensure that the meals are within your capabilities of making. It is important you eat right and keep to your fasting schedule. Your body is going to be switching to ketosis. This is accomplished much easier when you keep your diet and fast consistent.

Be prepared for the symptoms of the change. If you are knowledgeable, you will not be blindsided by the side effects. Keep electrolytes on hand, and if you need additional supplements such as magnesium, potassium, or sodium, have them on hand. The first week is the hardest! You got this.

If you are pairing this diet with exercise, take it easy. If your workouts are normally strenuous, try to be consistent. If you do not normally work out, do not overdo it. Slow and steady wins the race – and helps you get into a weight loss routine.

Week Two – Weigh yourself. Check out how much weight you lost in the first week and track it. You can do this in a multitude of ways. Some people prefer journals, apps, notebooks. Whatever works best for you – utilize it.

Re-evaluate if your fasting schedule is working for you. If it is, great! Keep going. If you find that it does not quite gel with your lifestyle, feel free to adjust, or switch to a different fasting method. If you make a change, remember that you need to try it out for the rest of the week. Keep changes as consistent as possible.

Stay strong on your keto! Make meaningful purchases when you buy food. Refer to the recipes in this book if you need some inspiration for what to cook and how to cater to yourself. The keto diet will really help give you the boost you need while fasting.

If you are on an exercise program, stay strong. Document your goals, take pictures! Use whatever motivates you. Remember, this journey is about your dreams and goals for yourself! You achieve those when you remain consistent and strong in your exercise and keto fasting.

Week Three – Get back on that scale! Celebrate in the successes that you have made. You should now be feeling the full effects of keto and fasting. Your body should be in a constant fat burning state. Good for you! You Made it.

If your fasting method needs adjusting, do it at the beginning of week three. You can do this adjustment weekly until you find a method that matches your needs. It is a versatile way to fast, so do not be shy to plan it into your life. It can take several tries before you find the perfect match.

Your keto diet should be in full swing as well. It should begin feeling familiar, manageable and you should also be feeling the benefits. There are many kinds of recipes that you can use in order to keep your keto meal plan diverse. Play around with recipes, try something new. You can also try a keto dessert! Yes, being on keto does not restrict you from dessert. Try one of the great dessert recipes in this guide.

Week Four – You should have four weeks of Keto fasting results by now. Look at the weight loss you have lost. Have you met your goals? Did you far surpass your goals? Do you see that inches and pounds have shredded off your waistline? Did you stick to your fasting schedules and keto diets?

Your health will be in its most optimal shape if you have successfully woven both keto and intermittent fasting into one lifestyle change. Remember for women that keto is necessary in order to safely reap all the benefits that intermittent fasting has to offer you. You gain only benefits when you pair them together.

At the end of week four, you will have all the results you need to see how successful these diets are together. It is hard to argue with results. So, see for yourself. I promise you will not be disappointed.

Time to Check In

This chapter was simple. It really is where you narrow down a thirty-day action plan that you can use to track your goals. Having an action plan keeps you accountable for where you are supposed to be on your weight loss journey.

It is not an overnight process, and it takes time to adjust to. Sometimes it can even take several different tries before you find a method that works best for you. The first 30 days are going to be about trial and error, but as long as you stick to your routine you will see results! Our goal is eight pounds in these first thirty days, I know you can lose more! So, set goals and limits – make sure they are attainable. If you set unrealistic goals, then you will only end up disappointing yourself. So, always make sure that your goals are manageable and realistic. There is nothing wrong with dreaming big if you do not end up discouraging yourself!

Chapter Eight: Hypnosis, Meditation, and Weight Loss

Losing Weight on Meditation

Weight loss is a journey, there is no denying that. Sometimes that journey can feel stressful. But what if there were peaceful ways to promote weight loss whilst you are intermittent fasting and on the keto diet?

Meditation has been proven to aid weight loss and keep stress levels down. I am not crazy! I promise. Stay with this chapter, there is a ton you still must learn!

Meditation is a practiced skill in which you try to find calmness and clarity. It has been proven to lower blood pressure and help manage stress. High stress levels are not good in general, particularly when you are trying to fast and diet. There have been several studies and quite a bit of research conducted on how meditation affects weight loss. These studies have proven that meditation improves both binge eating and emotional eating habits.

So, what does meditation look like for you and why should you try it? There are so many beneficial reasons to try meditation. It is hard to argue you why you should not try it. Life changes can be stressful, and it can be hard to break old habits and patterns. But what if there was a way you could break away from that stress? Meditation might be the perfect fit for you.

Like fasting, meditation can take on a host of different appearances. But they all have four staple things in common. To make the most out of your meditation, there are some guidelines to follow.

A meditation zone can be anywhere you choose, but it must be a quiet location. Too much outside noise will distract you from your focus. Your meditation zone can be your favorite chair, a walk you take alone, or even the extra five minutes you spend in your car while it is parked in the driveway. There are no limits to your possibilities here.

You might conjure up a cross-legged position when you think of meditation. Throw this stereotype right out the window where it belongs. You can assume any posture that is comfortable for you. This can be standing, sitting, lying down, or even walking. It does not matter what position you get into, as long as it is comfortable for you and you can focus while in it.

You do need to focus on one thing, but there are no limitations to what that one thing is. If you find it beneficial to focus on your breathing, then do it. If you focus on a specific word or phrase, that is okay too. You just need to be able to keep focus on that one thing (it cannot be something that causes you stress, though. Remember this is supposed to relax you).

Keep a positive and open attitude when meditating. Do not berate yourself if your mind wanders or your focus shifts. Having other thoughts while meditating is natural. The key is to keep bringing them back to your original point of focus (your breath, or the word that you chose to initially focus on.) This is where the key difference will come into play.

When meditating, do not focus on how long you are meditating for, but rather the impact the meditation has on you. If you manage to quiet your mind within one minute of meditation, then that is all you need. Your meditation will not replace your keto diet and fasting schedule. It will help promote a healthier attitude toward your fasting, aid in your weight loss goals by giving you a more positive attitude toward food, and curbing those unhealthy binges.

Hypnosis and Weight Loss

There you go with that look again. Listen, I know this might all sound a little odd to you right now. But hey! I bet so did intermittent fasting before you learned all about it. Have I steered your wrong yet? Stay focused on this chapter, receive it with an open mind. You never know, it might change your entire life.

At the risk of sounding like a broken record, hypnosis is not a substitute for your fasting and keto regime. No, it is an added tool to use in conjunction with your diet and exercise. So, why use it? Not only has it been proven to be effective, but much like the meditation methods, it can make your lifestyle changes easier to adjust to.

Generally, you need the help of a hypnotherapist to help you achieve the state of hypnosis that you need. What is the state of hypnosis? Essentially, it is a state of concentration and absorption – sort of trance-like.

How does hypnosis help you? Simple. When you are under the state of hypnosis, you become a much more suggestable person. Because your attention is highly focused you respond better to suggestions that modify your behavior. These suggestions are done by using repetitive verbal and mental images.

If you are an emotional eater or a stress eater then you should consider hypnosis. Alone, hypnosis is not very effective as a weight loss program. But – and pay attention to this – when paired with other dieting methods, hypnosis can help reinforce positive behavior patterns that lead to an increased loss of weight while dieting. The reason for this is because you are less likely to fall into patterns of overeating when your hypnosis has kept reinforcing to you that you do not need to eat.

Overeating can be a very hard habit to kick when you first start a new diet or lifestyle change. But it is a crucial habit to kick because it makes all the difference on your path to the best you. Essentially, all your hypnosis techniques should be leaving you with stronger willpower.

Throw out all the images that the media has taught you about hypnosis. They do not wave a clock in front of you to get you to fall into a zombified state. They promote your mind to go into a state of peace and calm. You are still present, but it is like your subconscious is taking a backseat. You can hear everything that is going on around you.

If you are uncomfortable with having someone do this to you, there are ways to self-hypnotize. All the methods prompt you to focus on something calming in order to get into a state where you feel almost "zoned out." Before you do this though, you need to write down everything that you hope to achieve. Write down positive reinforcing statements about food. Record yourself saying these affirmations and place it with the sounds that you know calm you (this can be rain falling, talking about your favorite place or any trigger that calms you). Play this recording when you want to self-hypnotize. Remember, the idea is to give you positive mental reinforcements about food and eating habits.

Time to Check In

I am positive that now you better understand the benefits of hypnosis and meditation when it comes to weight loss. Let us just go over the main points to make sure that these key ideas stick.

- Meditation and hypnosis can both be used to help instill positive reinforcements about food, weight loss, and managing your diet.

- Meditation has been proven to reduce binge eating and emotional eating.

- Sometimes when we are stressed, we tend to cling to food as an outlet. Meditation and hypnosis work to reinforce ideas that food is meant as fuel and not as an emotional outlet.

- You can meditate anywhere, and in any position that is comfortable to you. Meditation looks different to everyone. Just try to focus and be in a quiet area.

- Hypnosis can be done by a hypnotist or even by yourself at home. Find a method that you feel comfortable with and practice with it.

- Remember that these methods do not replace your diet, but instead, they support and reinforce your weight loss.

It can be confusing trying to understand what exercise programs are best for you, especially if you are not an avid exerciser already. That's okay, the next chapter focuses on what exercises are best for you to try!

Chapter Nine: Let's Get Exercising!

Exercising Makes All the Difference

You can still exercise while intermittent fasting. In fact, it is encouraged! Exercise helps you tone and helps prevent you from losing any muscle mass. We want to lose the unnecessary fat but keep our muscle mass.

Before you start exercising you need to know how to plan your meals around your exercise routine. Let us take cardio for example. You never want to do your cardio workout on a full stomach. Plan your meals for the night before and work out in the morning. If this does not work for you, then try to space out your cardio workouts when you know you are in the post-absorptive state of your fasting schedule.

Cardio, weight-lifting, and other exercises are all on the table. You just need to be prepared with your meals to compensate for the energy you need to expend for your exercise routine.

There are some key exercises geared toward weight loss that you can practice while keto fasting. They are simple and effective!

Interval training is a very effective method for weight loss.

What is this, you ask? Well, essentially the goal is to get your heart rate up and then down again before bringing it right back up. What this looks like is normally an intense workout, resting, and then more active working out. Many people combine this into a 30-minute program by pushing themselves for 1 minute, resting for 1 minute, and then pushing themselves again in exercise the next minute. Indoor cycling is also a popular method to try interval training with.

Running is an awesome way to exercise and lose weight! You can do cardio on a treadmill or just by jogging around the park! Remember that your goal is weight loss, so challenge yourself. Add hills to your run. If you are on a treadmill up that incline. Push yourself, break a sweat and keep working out. You want to keep burning those pounds off.

Try to incorporate yoga into your schedule. While it will not help shed those pounds, it will keep you nimble and your body supple to complete those other workouts that you need to get done. Yoga will encourage your balance and even improve your mental focus. So, it is a win-win situation all around.

Some people hate running and high-intensity workouts. There is nothing wrong with that. Especially if you are not an avid exerciser. It can be normal to think of adding exercise programs with dread. But swimming is a pastime that most people enjoy, and it just so happens to be an effective workout method. A couple of laps in the pool works out all your core muscles, and it is a fairly low impact method of exercising. Want an exercise tip for swimming? A good workout method would be to try to tread water for as long as possible. This works best in the deepest end of the pool. When you can no longer tread water, rest for around two minutes. After your rest, do 10 sets of 100 meters each set. Make sure that you rest for one to two minutes between each set. Your muscles will be nicely exercised by the time you get out of the pool.

Remember the days when the skipping rope was your best friend? Well, here is a chance to reacquaint yourself with an old friend. Jumping rope can be an awesome workout that will also help you maintain consistent weight loss.

The great thing about the skipping rope is that it is inexpensive, can be taken and used anywhere! A quick routine that will get your heart pumping follows:

- Do a light 3-minute warm-up skip with the rope.

- Go ahead and do 100 jumps. Remember that both your feet leave the floor at the same time.

- After this, take your jump rope and do an additional 100 jump rope sprints. Essentially all this means is that you pick up the pace of your skipping.

- Keep going back and forth between the second and

third step, slowly decreasing the jumps each time you do it. So, if you start at 100-100 then go down to 50-50 for the next set. 21-21 jumps after that and eventually 9-9 jumps.

If you already exercise a lot, try to incorporate your regular routines into your new schedule. Remember not to overexert yourself, and if you feel faint, put the exercise away and pick it up once you have adjusted your meal and exercise schedule.

Time to Check In

When you add exercises to your keto and fasting routine, you increase your weight loss exponentially. Not only that but you keep your body toned and fit whilst fasting.

- Exercise is important. Do not skimp out on it. If you are already a regular exerciser, keep it up. Do not lose your momentum.

- Interval training is the best way that you can lose weight while fasting. It involves getting your heartbeat up, a period of active resting and then getting your heart rate right back up.

- High-intensity training is a good option for interval

training, but your meals need to be planned carefully.

- Cardio training is one of the best methods you can use. But mix it up. Add some hills or steep inclines to your cardio workout. Remember that the goal is to push yourself.

- Swimming is another viable option. It works out all those core muscles and builds muscle mass.

- Do not count out the jump rope. It can be your best exercise partner yet. Also, an easy method that you can take with you wherever you go.

Whatever exercise method you decide on, make sure that you are not overworking yourself. There are tons of other methods and tricks to intermittent fasting. Read on to the next chapter to find out a little more about what can make your weight loss journey a little easier for you.

Chapter Ten: Tips, Tricks, and Hacks for Beginners

Shortcuts that Work

Intermittent fasting can take a while to adjust to. After all, it is an entirely new way of having to think and change your lifestyle habits. Sometimes we need a little help, and that is where this chapter comes into action. Pay attention to these simple tips that can make a huge difference to how much you enjoy making this lifestyle change!

Avoid all drinks that are artificially flavored. All those labels that say low sugar, zero sugar, and diet drinks? Yes, you need to ditch those – like yesterday. All these diet drinks are loaded with artificial sweeteners, and they are no good for you. Plus, the negative side effects are a stimulated appetite. That means you revert to overeating, and after all the work you have put in to get here you do not want to take more steps backwards. I am just going to say this once: beef up your water intake. Drink as much water as you can stand. If you are thirsty, always try to switch out the drink you were going to have with a glass of water. You will be thankful in the long run.

Fasting hours can be tough. If you plan it around your sleep at least for roughly eight hours of the fast, you are asleep. But what about the times you are awake? A good tip is to make sure that you are busy during hours that you are fasting. Keeping busy keeps your mind occupied. This way you will think less about the food that you are not eating. If you find yourself with nothing to do try taking a walk, running an errand you have been putting off, or picking up an old hobby you had once put away.

Sleeping is a good tool to keep in your arsenal. You want to get enough rest each night to make sure that your body's system has time to recuperate from the days exercise. Also, your metabolism and fat burning do not stop while you are sleeping. In fact, they tend to increase, so sleeping can improve the amount of fat you burn (this does not mean sleep all day, just that you get the rest you need).

Try to maintain low-stress levels. Remember that being overstressed can be a trigger for overeating. Meditation is a great way to relax, and if you are prone to stress, it can mean the difference between your fasting failing or succeeding.

The best tip I can give you is to be honest with yourself. You cannot eat during your fasting period, and the only person you cheat is yourself. So, stick to your own boundaries. Do not cave into temptations when they arise and stay strong.

Tips to Get into Ketosis

Sometimes you just need a few extra reminders about how to get into ketosis. Well, that is what I am here to do.

The main thing you need to do in order to get into ketosis is to severely limit your carb consumption! You cannot achieve ketosis unless your diet is extremely low in carbohydrates. Remember that ketosis relies on the ketone molecules, so your blood ketone levels need to be up. If you are eating carbs, you are raising your glucose levels, and this is counterproductive to ketosis.

Coconut oil is a must for your diet! Why? Because it contains fats that are known as medium-chain triglycerides (MCT). I know, more long-winded science words. But hey! They are important to know. You might be wondering why these fats are so important? Well, unlike other fats, these fats get a first-class ride straight to the liver. They quickly find their way to the liver to be converted into ketones.

I cannot stress enough how important consuming healthy fats is! This is the whole basis of the keto diet, and it will ensure that you are in nutritional ketosis. Keep an eye on your macronutrients, refer to the previous charts as needed to recalculate your daily macronutrient needs. As long as these are balanced, and you are meeting what you need in order to stay in peak metabolic shape, then you have nothing to worry about.

Time to Check In

Nothing beats old-fashioned leg work. So, while these tips and tricks might give you clues as to what you need to do best to maintain your ketosis, keep in mind that it still lies on your shoulders to ensure that you are following your fasting schedule and your ketogenic diet.

These tips are great to refer to if you forget what propels you into ketosis, or if you need to troubleshoot how to ensure your body is in the metabolic state that you want it to be in.

Chapter Eleven: The Do's and Don'ts of Intermittent Fasting

Frequently Asked Questions

What is intermittent fasting?

It is not a diet. Intermittent fasting is a plan in which you restrict the times that you consume food. The object is to spend more time fasting than eating so you can reach nutritional ketosis.

What is Ketosis?

Ketosis is a metabolic state where your liver converts your stored fat into ketone molecules. These ketone molecules replace glucose and provide you with energy.

Will fasting make me enter starvation?

No. If you follow your plan and keep up with your meals when you are allowed to eat then all you are doing is entering fat burning mode when you are fasting.

Is intermittent fasting safe?

Yes! Intermittent fasting is safe! Women need to take a more laid-back approach to intermittent fasting than men do. Therefore, I recommend that you pair your ketogenic diet and intermittent fasting together. This is the safest way to use fasting as a woman.

I am scared, is fasting right for me?

It is always a good idea to consult your doctor before making any major dietary or lifestyle changes.

Are there benefits to fasting?

In case you missed the benefits section, I am going to do two things here. First, I am going to refer you back to the introduction to intermittent fasting. A whole host of benefits are listed there! I promise you that I would not recommend intermittent fasting if there were no benefits to you. The other thing I will do is just provide you with a small list of the benefits you can expect to see with keto fasting.

- Fat loss

- Decreased insulin levels and decreased insulin resistance

- Decreased inflammation

- Good for your heart

- Increased energy and focus

- Keep muscle mass

What about the disadvantages?

There are studies that show women have a harder time adapting and benefiting to the intermittent fasting lifestyle. That is why I recommend that you also use to keto diet. If you pair keto and fasting together, you will remove the negative side effects of fasting. Also, keep in mind you need to take a more relaxed approach to fasting than a man.

Do's and Don'ts of Fasting

This one is simple. Do follow what I have set as guidelines for you here throughout this book.

Do pair your ketogenic diet with intermittent fasting.

Do count your macronutrients and ensure you are getting high fats, moderate proteins, and low carbs each day.

Do ensure that you are sticking to your fasting window.

Do clean out your kitchen of foods that are not good for you.

Don't listen to old wives' tales. Seek your doctor's opinions if you are concerned about myths that you hear.

Don't overload yourself. Take it one step at a time. Allow yourself to get comfortable and find out what works for you.

Don't cheat! The only person who loses when you cheat is yourself.

Chapter Twelve: Supporting Resources

Ketogenic Shopping List

Listen, I get it. Throwing out the contents of your cupboard can be scary. But that does not mean it is not manageable! Having a list of items to look out for that you can save and/or go out and restock your cupboards with is important. This chapter is all about setting you up for success! That is easier to do if you know where to start with food. Combining keto with intermittent fasting increases your weight loss percentage and other health benefits, but you need a list to take grocery shopping. That is where this comes in! So, buckle up, we have a few great shopping lists you can use when going keto!

Meat – always opt for grass-fed beef and pasture raised chicken and pork. Seafood should be wild caught and not farmed.

Fats make up around seventy-five percent of the average ketogenic diet. So, having access to healthy fats is extremely important. Omega 3 fatty acids have anti-inflammatory benefits, and so these are the fats we need to increase in our diets. Here is a quick list:

- Salmon

- Sardines

- Eggs

- Chia seeds

- Flax seeds

- Walnuts

- Cod liver oil

- Hemp seeds

- Grass-fed butter

There are also acceptable sweeteners that you can use while on the keto diet – remember that these need to be used in moderation.

- Stevia

- Monk fruit

- Erythritol

- Allulose

- Truvia

Vegetables are fair game if they are not starchy! There are way too many vegetables to list, but I will give you a great head start! Think broccoli, cauliflower, carrots, mushrooms, onions, cabbage, green beans, celery, brussel sprouts, beetroot, peas, artichokes, garlic, okra, rutabaga, and a host of other great veggies! There is so much you can do with vegetables you will never get bored!

Fruits are also fair game, but you do need to be a little more cautious with the kinds of fruits that you eat. Focus on these below:

- Berries (raspberries, strawberries, blueberries, blackberries)

- Avocado

- Coconut

- Peppers

- Cucumbers

- Tomatoes

- Lemon

- Lime

The amazing thing about the keto diet is that dairy is not forbidden! In fact, whole fats are encouraged. This adds great variety to our diets. So, a list of good dairy products would be:

- Butter

- Heavy whipping cream

- Cream cheese

- Sour cream

- Plain Greek yoghurt

- Cream

- Nut milks (like almond milk)

- Cottage cheese

You might be wondering about good pantry items to stock? Well clear that pantry out and make room for a host of options!

- Psyllium husk powder (if you are a baker or like bread this is a must stock in your pantry)

- Apple cider vinegar

- Balsamic vinegar

- Sea salts

- Dill pickles

- Bone broths

- Dried herbs

- Nuts and seeds

- Coconut milk and cream

These items should be stocked in your kitchen and are good for beginners just starting out on keto fasting! They will introduce you to the basics until you are more confident in your keto shopping!

Sometimes you just need a list of snacks that are okay to eat! Well, say no more. If you are more of a snacker, I have some great keto friendly ideas for you. Keep in mind that these can only be consumed during your eating window!

Here is a list of keto friendly and safe snacks that you can partake in without any extra feelings of guilt! Enjoy!

- A slice of ham that is spread with either mayonnaise or cream cheese. It can be wrapped up by itself or with a leaf of lettuce.

- Cooked bacon with tomato pieces and mayonnaise in a rolled-up lettuce leaf.

- Cooked steak, pork, or chicken diced into pieces and mixed in with avocado or cream cheese.

- Slices of smoked salmon and cream cheese.

- Smoked salmon and scrambled egg mixture, topped with cream cheese.

- Tuna mixed with mayo and cream cheese topped onto slices of cucumber.

- Olives stuffed with feta cheese.

- Baked chicken wings (do not add breading). Can use a blue cheese dressing with these.

- Celery stuffed with cream cheese.

What Can I Drink?

Let me first start by saying that you cannot eat anything outside of your eating window. But there are several things that you can drink during your fasting window. Water, coffee, broths, tea, and apple cider vinegar are all drinks that can be consumed throughout the day. There is no cap on the amount of water you can drink. Have it still or sparkling. Add some lemon or don't. Enjoy it the way you want!

Your coffee should ideally be black. Avoid adding sweeteners or milk as this is prohibited outside of your eating window.

Good news though, you can add spice to the coffee! So, cinnamon is okay.

Doing a twenty-four hour fast? Then you want to stock up on either a vegetable or bone broth. These are recommended during long fasts. Avoid broths from cans or bouillon cubes. Always go homemade if you can. A broth is an easy item to make ahead of time and store!

Remember to avoid those sugary drinks and the diet drinks! They are bad for you and do not qualify as a safe keto or intermittent fasting drink. Stick to the list provided, avoid high sodium contents and artificial sweeteners, and you will be golden!

Sweet Surprises

I know that I gave you a whole list of meals that you can use for breakfast, lunch, and dinner. But I just wanted to let you know that I am so proud of you for making it this far and sticking through this journey!

I really believe that you will benefit. As a thank you, I am enclosing some additional recipes. These recipes are for just desserts! Yes, you read that right. You can still enjoy a great dessert while keto fasting. Try your hand at a few of these, you cannot go wrong!

Keto Berry Mousse

Ingredients:

2 cups heavy whipping cream

3 ounces fresh raspberries, strawberries or even blueberries

2 ounces chopped pecans

½ lemon the zest

¼ tsp vanilla extract

Directions:

- Pour the cream into a bowl and whip it with a hand mixer until soft peaks form. You can use an old whip too, but this will take some time. Add the lemon zest and vanilla once you are almost done whipping the cream mixture.

- Combine berries and nuts into the whipped cream and stir it thoroughly.

- Cover the mousse with plastic wrap and let it sit in the refrigerator for 3 or more hours for a firmer mousse. If your goal is to have a less firm consistency, you can eat the dessert right away.

Cinnamon Crunch Balls

Ingredients:

  3 ounces unsalted butter

  ½ cup unsweetened shredded coconut

  ¼ teaspoon ground cardamom

  ½ teaspoon vanilla extract

  ¼ teaspoon ground cinnamon

Directions:

- Bring the butter to room temperature.

- Roast the shredded coconut carefully until they turn a little brown. This will create a delicious flavor, but you can skip this if you want. Let cool.

- Mix together butter, half of the shredded coconut and spices in a bowl.

- Form into walnut-sized balls with two teaspoons. Roll in the rest of the shredded coconut. Store in refrigerator or freezer.

Keto Cheesecake and Blueberries

Crust –

Ingredients:

  1¼ cups almond flour

  2 ounces butter

  2 tablespoons erythritol

  ½ tsp vanilla extract

Filling –

Ingredients:

  20 ounces cream cheese

  ½ cup heavy whipping cream

  2 eggs

  1 egg yolk

  1 teaspoon lemon, zest

  ½ tsp vanilla extract

  2 ounces fresh blueberries (optional)

Directions:

- Preheat the oven to 350 degrees F.

- Butter a 9-inch baking dish and line the base of it with parchment paper.

- Next, melt the butter for the crust and heat it until it lets off a nutty scent. This will give the crust an almost toffee-like flavor.

- Remove it from the heat and add the almond flour and vanilla. Combine these into a firm dough and press the dough into the base of the pan. Bake for about 8 minutes, until the crust turns lightly golden. Set the crust aside and allow it to cool while you prepare the filling.

- Combine cream cheese, heavy cream, eggs, lemon zest, and the vanilla. Combine these ingredients well and make sure there are no lumps. Pour this cheese mixture over the crust.

- Raise the heat of the oven to 400 degrees F and bake for another 15 minutes.

- Lower the heat to 230 degrees F and bake for another 45-60 minutes.

- Turn off the heat and let the dessert cool in the oven. Remove it when it has cooled completely and place it in the fridge to rest overnight. Serve it with fresh blueberries.

Keto Gingerbread Crème Brule

Ingredients:

1¾ cups heavy whipping cream

2 teaspoons pumpkin pie spice

2 tablespoons erythritol (an all-natural sweetener)

¼ teaspoon vanilla extract

4 egg yolks

½ clementine (optional)

Directions:

- Preheat the oven to 360 degrees F.

- Crack the eggs to separate them and place the egg whites and the egg yolks in two separate bowls. We will only use egg yolks in this recipe, so save the egg whites for a rainy day.

- Add some cream to a saucepan and bring to a boil along with the spices, vanilla extract, and sweetener mixed in.

- Add the warmed cream mixture into the egg yolks. Do this slowly, only adding a little bit at a time, while whisking.

- Pour it into oven-proof ramekins or small Pyrex bowls that are firmly placed in a larger baking dish with large sides.

- Add some water to the larger dish with the ramekins until it's about halfway up the ramekins. Make sure not to get water in the ramekins though. The water helps the cream cook gently and evenly for a creamy and smooth result.

- Bake in the oven for about 30 minutes. Take the ramekins out of the baking dish and let the dessert cool.

- You can enjoy this dessert either warm or cold. You can also add a clementine segment on top of it.

I bet you never thought that dieting could be so tasty! Think of all the wasted years trying methods that were tasteless and yielded no results. Are you not just so glad that you found this method? What about the food? Is your mouth watering at the prospect of all these meals that you get to eat while still safely staying within the boundaries of your keto fasting? I bet it is!

*** The recipes in this guide are all adaptations from recipes by Anne Aobadia. They do differ in ingredients and methods here and there, but they are still all tasty. These recipes are designed to give you the necessary macronutrients that you need to go about your day while intermittent fasting.

Conclusion

Congratulations! You made it all the way through. Do you know what this now means? It means that you are ready to start to conquer your journey to the best version of you! Everyone has their own ideal image for themselves, and using intermittent fasting and keto can get you there.

I am confident that you now have both the tools, the knowledge, and the action plan that will get you kick-started on this new lifestyle. Things might be difficult at the beginning, but your perseverance will make all the difference to you in this diet.

Remember that as a female it is important to pair intermittent fasting with the ketogenic diet. They go together like wine and chocolate – it is a no brainer. Both dietary lifestyles will complement each other so that you can receive the optimal benefit from both.

If you ever get stuck come back to the chapters that will get you moving again! Remember, you have the action plan, exercise routines, a shopping list, and even some meals all packed into this guide! It is completely up to you what you make of your weight loss journey from here. I wish you the utmost of luck as you embark on this lifestyle that leads to a path of mental and physical benefits.

References

Aobadia, A. (2018). Top Keto Meals – Delicious Recipes for Lunch & Dinner – Diet Doctor. Retrieved from https://www.dietdoctor.com/low-carb/keto/recipes/meals

Beginner Keto Grocery List. (2019). Retrieved from https://theketoqueens.com/beginner-keto-grocery-list/?cn-reloaded=1

Brooks, S. (2019). Why Keto Is More Effective with Intermittent Fasting. Retrieved from https://blog.bulletproof.com/keto-intermittent-fasting-weight-loss-diet/

Five Surprising Benefits of Meal Planning. (2018). Retrieved from https://www.mealplanmagic.com/blogs/meal-planning/five-surprising-benefits-of-meal-planning

Gunnars, K. (2015). 11 Myths About Fasting and Meal Frequency. Retrieved from https://www.healthline.com/nutrition/11-myths-fasting-and-meal-frequency#section10

Gunnars, K. (2016). 10 Evidence-Based Health Benefits of Intermittent Fasting. Retrieved from https://www.healthline.com/nutrition/10-health-benefits-of-intermittent-fasting#section9

Hamzic, H. (2019). Intermittent Fasting on Keto: How Does It Work? Retrieved from https://www.kissmyketo.com/blogs/foods-nutrition/intermittent-fasting-on-keto-how-does-it-work

Hicks, C. (2015). Why fasting is now back in fashion. Retrieved from https://www.telegraph.co.uk/lifestyle/11524808/The-history-of-fasting.html

Kodas, E. (2014). Meditation for Weight Loss: Emotional Eating, Mindfulness, and Awareness. Retrieved from https://www.webmd.com/balance/features/meditation-hypertension-and-weight-loss#2

Lefave, S. (2019). 10 of the Best Workouts for Weight Loss. Retrieved from https://www.self.com/story/10-insanely-effective-workouts-for-weight-loss

McLeod, C. (2018). The 6 people who shouldn't try intermittent fasting, according to a dietitian. Retrieved from https://www.bodyandsoul.com.au/nutrition/nutrition-tips/the-6-people-who-shouldnt-try-intermittent-fasting-according-to-a-dietitian/news-story/ca97f74fc904811f4b78281824dea72c

Schultz, R. (2018). Everything You Need to Know About the Benefits of Using Hypnosis for Weight Loss. Retrieved from https://www.womenshealthmag.com/weight-loss/a19937534/hypnosis-for-weight-loss/

Weighs, L. (2019). How Should You Exercise While You're Intermittent Fasting? Doctors Weigh In. Retrieved from https://www.mindbodygreen.com/0-29179/how-should-you-exercise-while-youre-intermittent-fasting-doctors-weigh-in.html

What Is Intermittent Fasting? Explained in Human Terms. (2019). Retrieved from

https://www.healthline.com/nutrition/what-is-intermittent-fasting#section3